A Model for Integrated Health, Child and

We would like to express a word of thanks to all who have supported the publication of this book, all co-authors for their efforts, the Dutch Federation of University Medical Centres (www.nfu.nl), Utrecht, The Netherlands; the Tjommie Foundation (www.tjommie.nl), Apeldoorn, The Netherlands; and the Royal Netherlands Embassy, Pretoria, South Africa, who all made it financially possible to write and publish this book.

Second print 2011
First print 2010

© 2010 The authors and VU University Press, Amsterdam

VU University Press is an imprint of
VU Boekhandel/Uitgeverij bv
De Boelelaan 1105
1081 HV Amsterdam
The Netherlands

Website: www.vu-uitgeverij.nl
E-mail: info@vu-uitgeverij.nl

ISBN 978 90 8659 477 1
NUR 870

Design cover: Titus Schulz, Arnhem
Type setting: JAPES, Amsterdam (Jaap Prummel)

A Model for Integrated Health, Child and Community Care in Rural South Africa

edited by

Hugo Tempelman
Mariette Slabbert
Anke Gosling
Adri Vermeer

in cooperation with

Geert Blijham: Preface
Frank Miedema: Epilogue
Alison Fisher: Copyeditor
&
Ndlovu Care Group Staff

Ndlovu Care Group
VU University Press
Amsterdam 2010

Correspondence Addresses

Mr. H.A. Tempelman, MD, MA
Ndlovu Care Group
P.O. Box 1508
Groblersdal 0470
South Africa
e-mail: tempelman@ndlovu.com

Mrs. M. Slabbert, MBA
Ndlovu Care Group
P.O. Box 1508
Groblersdal 0470
South Africa
e-mail: mariettes@ndlovu.com

Prof. A. Vermeer, PhD
Utrecht University
Faculty of Social and Behavioural Sciences
Department of Pedagogical and Educational Sciences
Heidelberglaan 1
3584 CS Utrecht
The Netherlands
e-mail: a.vermeer@uu.nl

Contents

Part Three
Community Services, the Community Health Awareness Mobilisation & Prevention Programme (CHAMP)

Epilogue

Preface

Holland is a rich country. Less than 5% of Dutch citizens live below the poverty line, and even this level may be considered "high" compared to what is labelled poor in other parts of the world. Holland also has an excellent health care system as documented by numerous international studies. In particular, there is virtually no access issue. Every Dutch citizen must be insured and is entitled to the best health care. Certainly, people do complain about waiting times, costs and quality, but in general, they all know that these are luxury complaints. How different is the situation in South Africa!

Dutch doctors and nurses have a long tradition of working in so-called developing countries, in particular in Africa. As a former president of one of the largest medical centers of The Netherlands, I can testify to this in two ways. Firstly, when appointing new professors it is amazing to see how many of them have spent some years in Africa. Apparently, the nation's talent feels deeply attracted to working in conditions that are completely different and certainly more challenging. Secondly and in line with that observation, Dutch university medical centers have been engaged in collaborations with medical projects and institutions in Africa quite extensively. We consider these collaborations fruitful at different levels: to expose our students to other disease diagnoses and health care systems, to maintain our doctors' skills that they otherwise might lose and to contribute to breakthroughs by our scientists that really matter. For UMCs, Africa is not a lost continent.

For these reasons, the presidents of the eight Dutch UMCs were very eager to see what our fellow countryman Hugo Tempelman has been doing in Elandsdoorn. So, on our annual journey to important medical places of common interest, we made our way to his HIV clinic, his maternity clinic, the community services, in short to all aspects of community health care that he, his collaborators and his services are offering. And we were so impressed that we started to think: how can we support the application of these approaches and these results to a larger audience, in fact to the world? I, as the acting chairman of the Federation of the eight Dutch UMCs, could easily convince my colleagues to come to a common and enthusiastic conclusion: we will support a book that describes what has been done and is going on in Elandsdoorn. That book is now lying in front of you.

For the University Medical Center Utrecht and Utrecht University, there is another reason to be excited about this book. For years, Hugo Tempelman has had special ties with those two Dutch institutions. As a visiting professor he has been instrumental in assisting the Faculty of Social and Behavioural Sciences to do groundbreaking research on the behavourial aspects of community health care programmes. In collaboration with the UMC Utrecht, very interesting data regarding HIV infections were obtained and published. Utrecht and Ndlovu: it has turned out to be an extremely successful collaboration between academia and community that deserves to be further developed and utilised.

The Ndlovu Care Group has grown upon the determination and stamina of a few in order to benefit the many. This book tells you the story. We as eight Dutch UMCs are proud to support the dissemination of that story. We hope it is as inspiring to you as it was to us.

Geert H. Blijham
Em. Professor of Medicine, UMC Utrecht/Utrecht University
Former president of UMC Utrecht
Chairman of Ndlovu Care Group Board of Trustees

List of Acronyms

ABCD: Asset Based Community Development
AIDA-model: Awareness/Attention Interest Desire Action-model
AIDS: Acquired Immunodeficiency Disease Syndrome
AIS: AIDS Indicator Surveys
AMREF: African Medical and Research Foundation
ANOVA: Analysis of Variance
ANC: African National Congress
ANC: Antenatal Care
APA: American Psychology Association
ART: Antiretroviral Treatment/Therapy
ARV: Antiretroviral
ASAP: As Soon As Possible
ATC: Autonomous Treatment Centre
AZT/3TC/NVP: HIV Therapy

BCEA: Basic Conditions of Employment Act
BCG drops: BCG vaccine
BCHC: Bhubezi Community Health Centre
BSS: Behaviour Surveillance Surveys

CCC: Community Care Community
CCMA: Commission for Conciliation, Mediation and Arbitration
CD4:   Cluster of Differentiation 4
CDC: Centre for Disease Control and Prevention
CEO: Chief Executive Officer
CFO: Chief Financial Officer
CHAMP: Community Health Awareness Mobilisation Prevention
CHC: Community Health Centre
CHET: Centre for Higher Education Transformation
CHW: Community Health Worker
CMC: Columbine Maternity Clinic
COIDA: Compensation for Occupational Injuries and Diseases Act
COO: Chief Operations Officer
CPSI: Centre for Public Service Innovation
CRC: Convention of the Rights of the Child
CSO: Civil Society Organisation
CV: Curriculum Vitae

DFID:	Department for International Developement
DHS:	Demographic & Health Surveys
DoH:	Department of Health
DOTS:	Direct Observed Treatment Support
DSMIV:	Diagnostic Statistical Manual IV
EB:	Executive Board
ECD:	Early Childhood Development
EEP:	Environmental Education Programme
EHR:	Electronic Health Record
EPTB:	Extra Pulmonary Tuberculosis
ETR:	Electronic Tuberculosis Record
FBO:	Faith-Based Organisation
FETI:	Further Education and Training Institute
FGASA:	Field Guides Association of Southern Africa
FHI:	Family Health International
FIFA:	Fédération Internationale de Football Association
FIFO:	First In First Out
FPD:	Foundation for People Development
GDP:	Gross Domestic Product
GP:	General Practitioner
GPP:	Good Pharmacy Practice
HAART:	Highly Active Antiretroviral Treatment
HBC:	Home-Based Care
HCT:	HIV Conselling and Testing
HDI:	Human Development Index
HIV:	Human Immunodeficiency Virus
HPV:	Human Papilloma Virus
HRM:	Human Resource Management
HSCR:	Human Sciences Research Council
HW Seta:	Health and Welfare Sector Education and Training Authority
ICCC:	Innovative Care for Chronic Conditions
ICD10:	International Classification of Diseases 10
ICESCR:	International Convenant on Economic, Social and Cultural Rights
ICF:	International Classification of Human Functioning
IDU:	Intravenous Drugs User
IEC:	Information, Education & Communication
IPT:	Isoniazid Preventative Therapy
IT:	Information Technology
IQ:	Intelligence Quotient
KAPP:	Knowledge Awareness Perception Practice

LBR act:	National Library of South Africa Act
L&D:	Learning & Development
LRA:	Labour Relations Act
MA:	Master of Arts
MAD:	Mobilise Awareness Destigmatise (campaign)
MANOVA:	Multivariate Analysis of Variance
MBA:	Master of Business Administration
MDG:	(United Nations) Millennium Development Goals
M&E:	Monitoring & Evaluation
MICS:	Multiple Indicator Cluster Surveys
MPB:	Mpumalanga Parks Board
MSc:	Master of Science
MSF:	Médicins Sans Frontières
MSM:	Men who have Sex with Men
MTCT:	Mother to Child Transmission
MTPA:	Mpumalanga Tourism & Parks Agency
NAAP:	Ndlovu AIDS Awareness Programme
NCCP:	Ndlovu CHAMP Children's Programme
NCG:	Ndlovu Care Group
NCP:	Ndlovu Children's Programme
NGO:	Non Governmental Organization
NHI:	National Health Insurance
NHLS:	National Health Laboratory Service
NHP:	Ndlovu HAART Project
NMA:	Ndlovu Music Academy
NMC:	Ndlovu Medical Centre
NNU:	Ndlovu Nutritional Unit
NPO:	Non Profit Organisation
NRC:	Ndlovu Research Consortium
NSAIDS:	Non-Steroidal Anti-Inflammatory Drugs
NSP:	National Strategic Plan
OVC:	Orphans & Vulnerable Children
PAP:	Papanicolau
PDD:	Project Design Document
PEP:	Post-Exposure prophylaxis
PEPFAR:	United States President Emergency Plan for AIDS Relief
PEST:	Practical Environmental Socio-Economic Technological
PHC:	Primary Health Care
PhD:	Doctor of Philosophy
PLWA:	People living with AIDS
PME&R:	Planning Monitoring Evaluation & Reporting
PMTCT:	Prevention of Mother To Child Transmission

PNC:	Postnatal Care Service
PR:	Public Relationship
PRA:	Participatory Rapid Appraisal
PPP:	Public Private Partnership
PTB:	Pulmonary Tuberculosis
RAP:	Rural Advancement Plan
RNE:	Royal Netherlands Embassy
SA:	South Africa
SACBC:	Southern African Catholic Bishops' Conference
SAMA:	South African Medical Society
SANAC:	South African National AIDS Council
SAPS:	South African Police Service
SARS:	South African Revenue Services
SAS:	Statistical Analysis Software
SAT:	Scholastic Assessment Test
SIDA:	French for AIDS
SME:	Small and Medium Enterprises
SPSS:	Statistical Package for Social Sciences
STD:	Sexually Transmitted Disease
STI:	Sexually Transmitted Infections
SUA:	Step-up Adherence programme
TB:	Tuberculosis
TBP:	Theory of Planned Behaviour
UIF:	Unemployment Insurance Fund
UMC:	University Medical Centre
UN:	United Nations
UNAIDS:	United Nations AIDS programme
UNDP:	United Nations Development Plan
UNFPA:	United Nations Population Fund
UNGASS:	United Nations General Assembly Special Session
UNICEF:	United Nations International Children's Emergency Fund
UNISA:	University of South Africa
UNITAID:	International programme for drugs against HIV/AIDS, Malaria & TB
UP:	University of Pretoria
USAID:	United States Agency for International Development
UU:	Utrecht University
VCT+:	Voluntary Counselling & Testing with CD4 staging and TB screening
WAZ:	Weight-for-Age Z-score

WHO:	World Health Organisation
WINMAX:	A tool for scientific text analysis
WWS:	Waterberg Welfare Society
XDR-TB:	Extremely drug-resistent tuberculosis
ZDV:	Zidovudine

Introduction

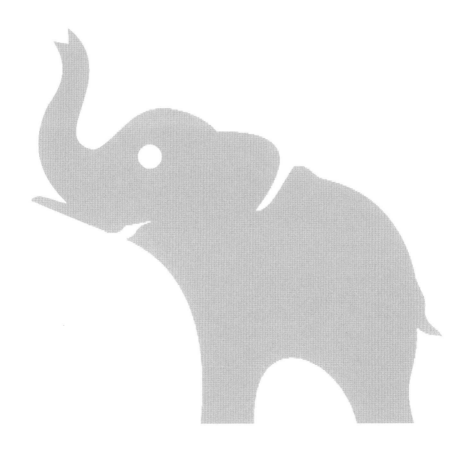

Perspectives of Health, Child and Community Care for the Advancement of Rural Areas in South Africa: An Introduction

Hugo Tempelman[a,b], Mariette Slabbert[c], Adri Vermeer[d]

1. Introduction

In the South African context, the majority of the population lives in poverty (Carter & May, 1999; Hargreaves, Morison, Gear, et al., 2007). The history of colonialism coupled with the legacy of apartheid have played a role in forming the current dualism which characterizes the South African social and economic class structure. This systemic dispossession has primarily affected the rural communities in South Africa.

Carter and May (1999) postulate that this has resulted in individuals in these communities having few assets aside from their own unskilled labor. This correlates with both Thurow's (1967) and Kozel and Parker's (2001) findings that poverty is the result of limited access to either one or a combination of resources, education and employment. Extrapolating from this, it is possible to assume that rural South Africans suffer from poverty of private assets as well as poverty of access to public goods and services.

2. Problem Statement

According to the Fact Sheet '*Poverty in South Africa, Human Sciences Research Council*' (Schwabe, 2004), estimates show that the proportion of people living in poverty in South Africa has not changed significantly between 1996 and 2001. However, those households living in poverty have sunk deeper into poverty, and the gap between rich and poor has widened.

South Africa has been a democratic state since 1994. Numerous programmes were initiated in an effort to improve the well-being of its citizens and address the imbalances of the past. The Human Sciences Research Council (HSCR) fact sheet states that in the past, inequality in South Africa was largely defined along race lines. It has become increasingly defined by inequality within population groups as the gap between rich and poor within each group has increased substantially, and the level of inequality is now comparable to that in the most unequal societies in the world.

---

a. CEO Ndlovu Care Group, Groblersdal, South Africa
b. Visiting Professor, Faculty of Social and Behavioural Sciences, Faculty of Medicine, Utrecht University, The Netherlands
c. COO Ndlovu Care Group, Groblersdal, South Africa
d. Professor emeritus of Special Education, Faculty of Social and Behavioural Sciences, Utrecht University, The Netherlands

Despite the following policy developments by the South African government, little has changed in the rural areas since 1994:
- Announcement of a 'War on Poverty' in the 2008 State of the Nation Address;
- Launch of the government's Draft Anti-Poverty Strategy;
- Public debate over a national poverty line;
- Proposals for a comprehensive social security system.

Some of the findings in the report, *Towards a 15-year review*, published by the SA government are that poverty remains a major challenge for South Africa and that there are serious inequalities in human social capital and major concerns over basic service delivery. The same report cites the following recommendations for an improved future:
1. reduce unemployment;
2. overcome structural causes of poverty and inequality;
3. 'pro-poor growth' plus 'pro-growth poverty reduction';
4. enhance social capital;
5. improve access to education and skills development.

The Department of Provincial and Local Government's Framework for a Municipal Indigent Policy (2005) states that it is now widely accepted that the experience of poverty is multi-dimensional. While the inability to access income remains one of the most obvious expressions of poverty, its definitions typically refer to the absence of capital such as land, the access to natural resources, or the importance of social and intellectual capital and even the climate of democracy and security necessary to enhance the capabilities of the poor and excluded. The social, environmental, political and economic dimensions of poverty are all relevant to local government, therefore. In South Africa, there is an additional institutional dimension of poverty that has rarely been addressed. The poorest in the nation are those who are unable to access state assistance designed to provide a social safety net because of institutional failure. Alongside the persistence of a second economy, the marginalization of the poor from the core administrative or institutional systems and resources of government is one of the key dimensions of persistent and chronic poverty. It is also known that these households in absolute poverty are geographically concentrated in townships, informal settlements and marginalized rural areas. The same report goes further: 'What is of concern here, however, is that economic exclusion has resulted in exclusion from access to basic services by the poor which contributes substantially to their experience of poverty'.

The underserved areas in which NCG operates, like Moutse East, Lesideng and Bushbuck Ridge, have limited access to essential household services like running water, waste removal, electricity, access to healthcare and sanitation. Unemployment and poverty are rampant, and schooling, although available, is often sub-standard and under-resourced.

While South Africa is amongst the 50 wealthiest countries in the world, with per capita GDP of $11,240 per annum in 2001, performance in terms of human development has been very poor. On the Human Development Index (HDI), SA ranked 115 out of 175 countries, a significant decline from the rank of 93 in 1992 (UNDP, 2003).

Approximately 57% of individuals in South Africa were living below the poverty income line in 2001, a level unchanged from 1996. Limpopo and the Eastern Cape had the highest proportion of poor with 77% and 72%, respectively, of their populations living below the poverty income line. In Mpumalanga it is 57% .The Western Cape had the lowest proportion (32%), followed by Gauteng (42%). This results in a GINI coefficient of 0.77 for South Africa, one of the worst in the world (Schwabe, 2004). 48% of the population of South Africa is below 18 years of age.

This disparity shows the inequity of South Africa. If we are unable to bridge this gap, the instability and social imbalance will remain to handicap the social transformation that South Africa deserves to undergo.

It is our opinion that the perception of too many donors and foreign governments that South Africa can be considered a middle-income country is wrong. With a GDP of $11,240 and 57% of the population living below the poverty line, retraction of donor support and development aid will set South Africa's development back tremendously. A country that has shown its ability to avert a civil war after the 1994 changeover deserves more support in the time they need it the most: the consolidation phase of the new democracy.

Woolard and Leibbrandt (1999) conducted a study of poverty levels in South Africa using household survey data. Their study included an analysis and discussion on identifying the poor, establishing a poverty line and profiling poverty in South Africa based on the outcomes. They concluded that the poor in South Africa are likely to be black and living in rural areas. In addition, they tend to have low levels of education and no access to wage employment or basic services including healthcare and transport. Furthermore, they are likely to be female-headed households (Woolard & Leibbrandt, 1999). Their findings are summarized in terms of the poverty profile outlined in their study as follows:

- *Location of the identified poor:* 63% poverty rate in rural areas compared with 22% in urban areas.
- *Poverty rates across racial lines:* Africans and coloureds show the highest rates of poverty at 51% and 30%, respectively, versus 3.1% amongst the remainder of the population.
- *Poverty differences across genders:* The poverty rate amongst female-headed households was 60% compared with 31% in male-headed households.
- *The relationship between poverty and education:* Findings indicate that the lower the level of education, the higher the rate of poverty, with a rate of 68% amongst those with no education versus 8.7% amongst those with tertiary education.
- *Health status and poverty:* Findings are specific to certain illnesses including tuberculosis, diarrhoea, fever, and physical and mental disability. On average, the incidence of these illnesses is twice as high as that for the total population. HIV/AIDS was not mentioned specifically in this study.
- *Employment and income among the poor:* The overall rate of unemployment in poor households is 52% compared with the national average of 29%. These figures largely correlate with the overall poverty profile.
- *The ability of the poor to access public goods and services:* Electricity, sanitation and piped water impact the quality of life, and findings show that a lack of access is closely linked to poverty.

- *Poverty and access to transportation:* Largely without access to public transportation, the working poor spend significant amounts of time and income on transportation, with the majority choosing to walk to work.

Furthermore, the HSRC report notes that it is commendable that South Africa is finally making progress against a number of indicators that are vital for an effective response to the AIDS epidemic. However, the report states that there are a number of areas requiring serious attention:
- HIV remains disproportionately high among women compared with men, and it peaks in the 25–29 age group, where one in three (32.7%) were found to be HIV-positive in 2008. This proportion has remained unchanged and was at the same level all the time.
- HIV is more than twice as high in women than in men in the age groups 20–24 and 25–29. HIV prevalence among men peaks in the 30–34 age group, where a quarter (25.8%) were found to be HIV-positive in 2008.
- Among youth, early sexual debut is related to sexual activity and consequent vulnerability to HIV infection. Sexual debut before the age of 15 among males aged 15–24 years declined from 13.1% in 2002 to 11.3% in 2008, but among females 15–24 years, 8.9% had had sex before the age of 15 in 2002, with 8.5% reporting the same in 2008.
- There was a substantive increase among young people who reported having partners more than five years older than themselves, from 9.6% in 2005 to 14.5% in 2008. The same pattern was also found among women, where the percentage increased substantively from 18.5% in 2005 to 27.6% in 2008.
- Having a high turnover of sexual partners influences the likelihood of exposure to HIV. Among people aged 15–49, the number of sexual partners reported in the past year has increased slightly since 2002, where 9.4% reported two or more partners in comparison with 10.6% in 2008.

According to the same report, HIV prevalence in the total population of South Africa has stabilized at a level of around 11%. However, HIV infection levels differ substantially by age and sex and also show a very uneven distribution among the nine provinces.

It is against this background that NCG finds its motivation: the inequity of South Africa and the tremendous disparity of how wealth is divided amongst a selected group while the overall population lives in deep poverty.

3. Aim and Outline of the Book

Ndlovu Care Group wants to replicate and prove its model for social mobilization through integrated Community Health & Community Care Services in underserved communities in South Africa. NCG wants to do this through its Rural Advancement Plan (RAP) that is the subject of this book.

Replication, by implication, requires that the services of NCG as an NGO are well described. To some extent, this is done by means of internal documents that are not publically available in one integrated volume. And thus, the first aim of this book becomes evident: to provide a systematic overview of the vision, mission, aims and programmes of NCG. This makes it clear which content NCG would like to replicate and the organizational structure behind this content. In this way NCG provides a picture about its services to the recipients of these services. Besides, NCG as an NGO is financially dependent on external donors to a great extent. By providing a systematic description of their starting points, strategies and programmes, NCG gives a responsible answer to questions about 'what return do donors receive on their investment?'.

The NCG organizational structure is based on two main divisions. First, the NCG Clinical Services, run by the Autonomous Treatment Centre (ATC), and second, the Community Services, run by the Community Health Awareness Mobilisation & Prevention (CHAMP) Programme. These two services are supported by a third division, the NCG Support Services. This structure is described and explained in the introductory *Chapter 1* (Tempelman & Slabbert) of *Part One*, The Ndolovu Care Group Model. Next, the services which are developed within the framework of the two divisions are described in *Part Two*, Clinical Services, The Autonomous Treatment Centre (ATC), and *Part Three*, Community Services, The Community Health Awareness Mobilisation & Prevention (CHAMP) Programme.

Replication also implies that NCG can rely on evidence-based results to prove the potential effectiveness, impact, and efficiency of the NCG model in rural settings. The NCG programmes operate on three different levels: community, household and individual levels that represent all age groups in a community. Research activities on all these levels ensure that NCG can prove that it achieves its objectives and demonstrate the extent to which the objectives are achieved. Research outcomes are used to improve the monitoring and evaluation of the programmes, adapt strategies, and localise and align indicators with the Millennium Goals and the SA National Strategic Plans of the various government departments. Research outcomes are also used to share experiences, contribute to the academic field and prove the effectiveness of the NCG RAP model.

To fulfil these goals, monitoring and evaluation procedures, described in *Part One, Chapter 4* (Kodisang), and evidence-based research procedures, described in *Part One, Chapter 5* (Gosling & Vermeer), are considered as belonging to the strategic development of NCG. The outcomes of these strategies contribute to the validation of the NCG programmes and, in turn, underpin the claim that the NCG model is replicable and transferrable.

Finally, before such evaluation activities can be carried out, the aims and methods of a specific programme to be evaluated have to be clearly described. If the kind of goals a programme is aiming at is not clear, it is not possible to determine and describe its outcomes. In *Part One, Chapter 6* (Vermeer), a frame of reference is provided for a programme description. By means of such a programme description, it is possible to evaluate the content and the internal consistency of a programme and to compare similar programmes with each other. This frame of reference can also be used for the monitoring and evaluation of the NCG programmes.

4. Conclusion

Ndlovu Care Group has achieved many of its objectives in the sites where it functions. This convinced us that we have developed a model for rural advancement that would benefit similar communities across South Africa. A model that we wanted to write down and share with those working in the same fields and for the same causes in order to contribute towards the closure of the poverty and treatment gaps in South Africa. That model is described in the book that lies in front of you.

References

Carter, M.R., & May, J. (1999). Poverty, livelihood and class in South Africa. *Elsevier, 27*, 1-20.

Hargreaves, J.R., Morison, L.A., Gear, J.S.S., Makhubele, M.B., Porter, J.D.H, Busza, J., Watts, C., Kim, J.C., & Pronyk, P.M. (2007). "Hearing the Voices of the Poor": Assigning Poverty Lines on the Basis of Local Perceptions of Poverty. A Quantitative Analysis of Qualitative Data from Participatory Wealth Ranking in Rural South Africa. *World Development, 35*, 212-2129.

Kozel, V., & Parker, B. (2001). *Poverty in Rural India: the Contribution of Qualitative Research in Poverty Analysis.* Washington DC: Poverty Reduction and Economic Management Unit, South Asia Region, World Bank.

Schwabe, C. (2004). Fact Sheet: Poverty in South Africa. Pretoria: *Human Sciences Research Council (HSRC).*

Thurow, L.C. (1967). The Causes of Poverty. *The Quarterly Journal of Economics, 81*, 39-57.

United Nations Development Programme (UNDP) (2003). *The World Resources Report 2002-2004: Decisions for the Earth: Balance, voice and power.* Global: UNDP, UNEP, World Bank, World Resources Institute.

Woolaard, I., & Leibbrandt, M. (1999). *Household Incomes, Poverty and Inequality in a Multivariate Framework.* University of Cape Town, Development Policy Research Unit, Working Papers Series, 1-27.

Part One

The Ndlovu Care Group Model

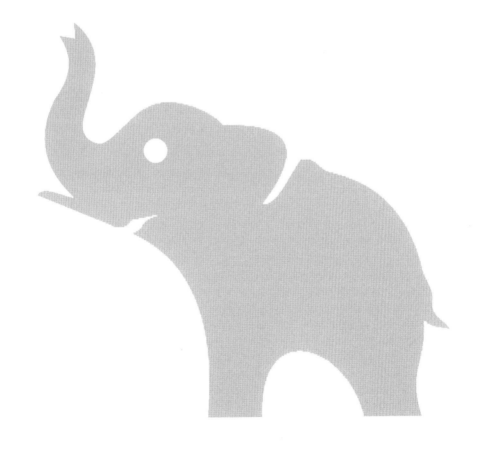

Chapter 1

The NCG Model for the Advancement of Rural Areas in South Africa

Hugo Tempelman[a,b], *Mariette Slabbert*[c]

Abstract

Ndlovu Care Group (NCG) wants to replicate and develop its model for social mobilisation through integrated Community Health & Community Care Services in underserved rural communities in South Africa by means of its Rural Advancement Plan (RAP). NCG wants to 'copy and paste' the RAP model to similar sites where there is no or only limited access to service delivery to assist the government in closing the existing 'treatment and poverty gaps' in these areas. NCG aligned its vision, mission, and objectives with the Millennium Development Goals (United Nations, 2002), the National HIV & AIDS and STI Strategic Plan for South Africa 2007-2011 (NSP 2007-2011, Department of Health [DoH], 2007), the national strategic plans of other government departments (Education, Arts & Culture, Home Affairs, etc.) and the Three Ones Strategy defined by the major donor organisations. Through public private partnerships (PPPs) with the relevant government departments, institutional donors, corporate institutions, and private investors, NCG wants to illustrate that the sustainable solution for uplifting rural populations lies in effective and appropriate collaboration amongst all sectors. The group has existed since 1994 and currently manages three RAP sites in South Africa: NCG Ndlovu in Moutse East (Limpopo Province), NCG Bhejane in Vaalwater (Limpopo Province) and NCG Bhubezi in Bushbuckridge (Limpopo Province). A fourth site, NCG Nyathi in Utah (Mpumalanga), is nearing completion and will be operational in 2010.

1. Introduction

NCG was founded in 1994 by Hugo Tempelman, a Dutch medical doctor, and his wife Liesje, a professional nurse. What started as a private general practice has since expanded to a corporate non-profit organisation (NPO) employing more than 240 people and operating in three locations, NCG Ndlovu in Moutse East (Limpopo Province), NCG Bhejane in Vaalwater (Limpopo Province) and NCG Bhubezi in Bush-

---

a. CEO Ndlovu Care Group, Groblersdal, South Africa
b. Visiting Professor, Faculty of Social and Behavioural Sciences, Faculty of Medicine, Utrecht University, The Netherlands
c. COO Ndlovu Care Group, Groblersdal, South Africa

buckridge (Limpopo Province). NCG integrates the delivery of primary health care, TB/HIV/AIDS care, child care and community development programmes to achieve its aim of advancing rural populations.

Achievements and growth of Ndlovu Care Group in chronological order:

1994 Start and opening of Ndlovu Medical Centre, a township-based community general practice.

1996 Opening of 1st Ndlovu Nutritional Unit and preschool in Moutse East.

1997 Start of Ndlovu Tuberculosis Programme in cooperation with provincial and national Departments of Health.

1998 Start of Ndlovu AIDS Awareness Programme.

1999 Opening of Maternity and 24-hour Clinic.

1999 Opening of Elandsdoorn Bakery.

2001 Opening of 2nd Ndlovu Nutritional Unit & Preschool.

2001 Opening of 1st water project in Lesehleng, Moutse East. NCG currently has 37 operational water projects in the area.

2001 Expanding Ndlovu Tuberculosis Programme with defaulter tracing.

2001 Start of Ndlovu Information Technology Training; community computer literacy programme.

2002 Opening of 3rd Ndlovu Nutritional Unit & Preschool in Thabachabedu, Moutse East.

2003 Start of mobile Community Dental Care Programme.

2003 Expanding Ndlovu Tuberculosis Programme with contact tracing and community TB Awareness.

2003 Start of Ndlovu Highly Active Anti-Retroviral Therapy (HAART) programme, a donor-funded ARV roll-out programme; the programme has over 7,000 patients enrolled for treatment and cares for around 12,000 HIV+ individuals.

2003 Construction of the first decentralised HIV monitoring laboratory in Moutse East.

2003 Start of Prevention of Mother to Child Transmission (PMTCT) programme with triple therapy, regardless of CD4 count levels, as a gold standard.

2003 Start of Waste Care Programme in Moutse East.

2004 Opening of 4th Ndlovu Nutritional Unit & Preschool in Phooko, Moutse East.

2004 Start of mobile HAART project for farmworkers (Mpumalanga and Gauteng).

2004 Opening of sport grounds in Moutse East.

2004 Start of Environmental Awareness and Education Childcare Programme in Loskop Nature Reserve, over 20,000 children have visited the reserve since 2004.

2005 Start of community Voluntary Counselling and Testing(VCT) programme.

2005 Start of Nappy Factory in Moutse East as a small business enterprise.

2006 Start of Orphans & Vulnerable Children (OVC) Programme; currently 3,500 children enrolled.

2007 Opening of 1st ATC satellite site at Vaalwater (Waterberg Welfare Society).

| 2007 | Opening of Bhubezi Community Heath Centre (BCHC) and Bhubezi AIDS Awareness Programme, Bushbuckridge, Limpopo Province |

2007   Opening of Bhubezi Community Heath Centre (BCHC) and Bhubezi AIDS
        Awareness Programme, Bushbuckridge, Limpopo Province
2008   Creation of NCG head office team to reposition NCG as a corporate NGO
        with professional support services that include monitoring & evaluation,
        finance, human resources, epidemiology, information technology, training
        and development, central procurement, and marketing & communications.
2008   Opening of the 'Miracle' Elandsdoorn, amphitheatre and start of the music
        academy.
2008   Receipt of Platinum Impumelelo Award for Innovation: Strengthening the
        Public Sector Service Delivery.
2008   Receipt of gold & silver CPSI awards for innovation and public-private
        partnership.
2009   Establishing Ndlovu Youth Choir.
2009   HAART programmes accredited with DoH.
2009   Completion of construction of NCG Nyathi Community Health Centre.
2010   Preschools accredited with DoH & Social Development.
2010   Receipt of Impumelelo 2010 Sustainability Award: Social Entrepreneur of the
        Year Award

2. NCG Alignment with National & International Plans

2.1. The Millennium Development Goals

The Millennium Development Goals (MDGs) are eight global goals to be achieved by 2015 that correspond with the world's main development challenges. The MDGs are drawn from the actions and targets contained in the United Nations Millennium Declaration that was adopted by 191 nations and signed by all heads of state and governments during the UN Millennium Summit in September 2002 (Sachs, 2005; p. 25):

- Eradicate extreme poverty & hunger
- Achieve universal primary education
- Promote gender equality & empower women
- Reduce child mortality
- Improve maternal health
- Combat HIV/AIDS, malaria, etc.
- Ensure environment sustainability
- Develop a global partnership for development

The eight MDGs break down into 21 quantifiable targets that are measured by 60 indicators.

The MDGs:
- synthesise, in a single package, many of the most important commitments made separately at the international conferences and summits of the 1990s;
- explicitly recognise the interdependence between growth, poverty reduction and sustainable development;

- acknowledge that development rests on the foundations of democratic governance, the rule of law, respect for human rights, and peace and security;
- are based on time-bound and measurable targets accompanied by indicators for
  monitoring progress; and
- bring together, in the eighth Goal, the responsibilities of developing countries with
  those of developed countries, founded on a global partnership endorsed at the
  International Conference on Financing for Development in Monterrey, Mexico,
  in March 2002, and again at the Johannesburg World Summit on Sustainable Development in August 2002.

If we superimpose the MDGs on the holistic approach of the Ndlovu Care Group
service delivery system, it follows that the NCG strategy could serve as a replicable
model to achieve localised implementation of most of the MDGs in a resource-poor
setting at the community level.

2.2. The National Strategic Plan

The HIV & AIDS and STI Strategic Plan for South Africa 2007-2011 (NSP 2007-2011)
flows from the National Strategic Plan (NSP) of 2000-2005 as well as the Operational
Plan for Comprehensive HIV and AIDS Care, Management, and Treatment for
South Africa. It represents the country's multi-sectoral response to the challenges
associated with HIV infection and the wide-ranging impact of AIDS.
   The primary aims of the NSP 2007-2011 are to:
- reduce the number of new HIV infections by 50%;
- reduce the impact of HIV and AIDS on individuals, families, communities and
  society by expanding access to appropriate treatment, care and support to 80% of
  all people diagnosed with HIV.

The interventions needed to reach the NSP 2007-2011's goals are structured under
four key priority areas:
- prevention;
- treatment, care and support;
- human and legal rights; and
- monitoring, research and surveillance.

The NCG Rural Advancement Plan (RAP) includes the NCG Community Health
Awareness, Mobilisation & Prevention (CHAMP) Programme, the NCG Autonomous Treatment Centre (ATC), the NCG Monitoring & Evaluation (M&E) activities
and the Research Consortium and covers all aspects addressed in the NSP 2007-2011.
The human and legal rights aspects are not covered as a separate programme but are
embedded at a variety of levels, e.g. gender issues, access to grants and official documentation, People Living With Aids (PLWA) support programmes, destigmatisation,
and inclusion of PLWA throughout all programmes. NCG adheres to and respects
human and legal rights.

2.3. The 'Three One's'

On 25 April 2004, the representatives of major donor organisations and of many developing countries adopted three principles as the overarching framework to improve coordination of the scale-up of national AIDS programmes and related responses to the HIV & AIDS epidemic. The 'Three Ones' are:
- *One* agreed HIV/AIDS *action framework* that provides the basis for coordinating the work of all partners;
- *One* national AIDS *coordinating authority*, with a broad-based, multi-sector mandate; and
- *One* agreed-upon country-level monitoring and evaluation system.

The importance of creating, implementing, and strengthening a unified and coherent Monitoring & Evaluation (M&E) system at the country level cannot be overemphasised. In South Africa the Departments of Health and SANAC (South African National AIDS Council; see Survey 2008), together with other relevant stakeholders, are responsible for the development and implementation of this national frame of reference.

There is the risk that separate disease- and donor-driven M&E systems will not have common data standards, compatible IT systems or reporting platforms. Coordination of the overall M&E system across a country is an important first step in building a common M&E system which can meet a variety of needs. In addition, many countries rely on surveys such as the Demographic and Health Surveys (DHS), AIDS Indicator Surveys (AIS), Multiple Indicator Cluster Surveys (MICS) and/or Behavioural Surveillance Surveys (BSS) that are funded through external donors. This produces data that may be valuable in the broader M&E context but may not be well integrated with traditional sources of health information, such as national health information and surveillance systems.

Although developed for AIDS, the principles have general relevance for M&E. By bringing together indicators for the three diseases (TB, HIV/AIDS, Malaria), the aim is to extend the 'Three Ones' beyond HIV to all three diseases (WHO, 2006; p. 8).

A strong and unified M&E system ensures that:
- relevant, timely, and accurate data are made available to national programme leaders and managers at each level of the programme and health care system;
- selected quality data can be reported to national leaders; and
- the national programme is able to meet donor and international reporting requirements under a unified global effort to contain the HIV/AIDS pandemic.

NCG agrees and adheres to the 'Three Ones' as far as they are formulated for South Africa: the NSP 2007-2011 is adhered to, the National M&E system is implemented, and NCG reports accordingly. NCG also aligns its operations to support the objectives of relevant government departments. A NGO's role is to assist the government in its efforts to implement strategic plans and to avoid setting up parallel systems out of frustration or paternalisation. Symbiotic cooperation with the government guarantees the sustainability and value of NGO programmes. Donors typically intervene in emergencies and do not intend to sustain countries in the long term, and it is therefore imperative that NGOs utilise donor funding as a means and not as an end in itself. The cooperation between the DoH and NCG, with the implementation of the Tuberculosis Programme in Moutse since 1997, demonstrates NCG's early efforts to integrate services and to strengthen government delivery. The successful accreditation of NCG in Limpopo Province (2009), as the first NGO for HIV-related services in that province, confirms NCG's efforts to make its programmes sustainable through integration into the public sector service delivery systems. In the same year the accreditation was achieved as well in Mpumalanga province.

3. The NCG Care Model

In NCG's 16 years of experience, there has been little improvement in the daily existence of the average township inhabitant in rural South Africa. High unemployment rates, migration for job opportunities, low levels of education, marginal service delivery at all levels in the townships, absent or dysfunctional family structures, high dependency on the social grant system for survival: all these factors maintain the inequality and inequity. The double epidemic of tuberculosis and HIV/AIDS hit South Africa much harder than surrounding countries and contributed in a horrific way to increasing the burden on the government to supply basic services in resource-poor settings. The overstretching of the health care services, the number of teachers who died, the increasing numbers of orphaned and vulnerable children (OVC), and the child-headed households all contribute towards stunting development and progress.

Furthermore, this situation negatively affected the confidence of the average inhabitant on the lower rungs of the economic ladder in the government's ability to improve service delivery.

Given this situation and the plight of the underserved areas, there is a need for NGOs, and this is why NCG took the initiative to adopt 'Empowering towards Wellness' as its vision. It is NCG's aim to strengthen the district systems and regain the trust and confidence of the rural populations through the delivery of quality health care services. NCG complements community health efforts with childcare programmes and community development programmes to uplift rural populations through motivation and by instilling a future orientation.

NCG achieves this through asset-based community development (ABCD), which involves cooperation with other non-governmental organisations (NGO), civil society organisations (CSO), corporations, and relevant government departments in its target areas. The NCG objective is to advance rural communities through prevention and motivation strategies that scale up services and develop skills and abilities in these communities.

NCG developed the RAP Care Model for service delivery in rural communities at the primary, secondary, and tertiary prevention levels.

Primary prevention is the prevention of diseases and conditions before their onset. Thus, general environmental and sanitary measures, such as maintaining a safe water and food supply, promoting the use of condoms to prevent sexually transmitted diseases, and application of safe and effective vaccines are examples of primary prevention, whereby diseases and injuries do not gain a foothold in the body.

Secondary prevention generally consists of the identification of diseases or conditions that are present but have not progressed to the point of producing signs, symptoms, and dysfunction. Disease screening (and follow-up of the findings) most often detects these preclinical conditions. Examples of screening procedures that lead to the prevention of disease emergence include VCT+ (Voluntary Counselling & Testing with CD4 staging and TB screening), the PAP smear for detecting early cervical cancer, routine mammography for early breast cancer, periodic determination of blood pressure and blood cholesterol levels, and screening for diabetes.

Tertiary prevention generally consists of preventing disease progression and suffering after it is clinically obvious and a diagnosis established. This activity also includes the rehabilitation of disabling conditions. Examples include eliminating offending allergens from asthmatic patients; routine screening for and management of early renal, eye, and foot problems among diabetics; preventing the reoccurrence of a heart attack with anti-coagulant medication and physical modalities to regain function among stroke patients and early intervention with anti-retroviral treatment for advanced HIV. For many common chronic illnesses, protocols to promote tertiary preventive interventions have been developed; they are often called 'disease management'.

This prevention approach aims at:
– preventing disease and adverse conditions from occurring;
– early detection of underlying disease and socio-economic challenges;
– minimisation of morbidity and mortality.

The RAP approach identifies and demarcates target areas and then educates the local population to take responsibility for the welfare of the community. RAP aims at:
– Local capacity building for sustained community development, improved employability and standard of living.
– Information, awareness, and education on health and development-related issues to promote behaviour change, early detection, early care-seeking behaviour and fewer new HIV infections.
– Affordable and integrated primary health care (PHC), malaria, TB and HIV/AIDS care to promote personal well-being and community health in general.
– Childcare programmes to address the needs and develop the life skills of orphans and other vulnerable children (OVC).
– Improved community service delivery, community development, entrepreneurial skills training and micro-lending.
– Evidence-based interventions through research, monitoring & evaluation to ensure improved outcomes.
– A replicable model for establishing health and community systems across rural areas in southern Africa.

In Figure 1 the organizational design of the Ndlovu Care Group and its services is shown.

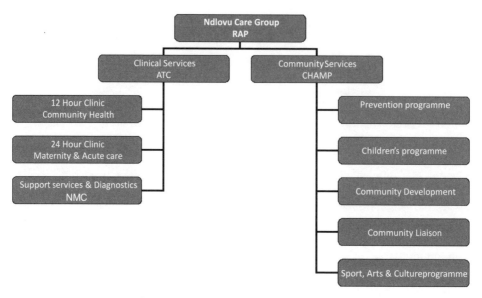

Figure 1: The organizational design of NCG and its services

4. The NCG Rural Advancement Plan

The NCG Rural Advancement Plan (RAP) consists of the Autonomous Treatment Centre (ATC) and Community Health Awareness Mobilisation & Prevention (CHAMP) programmes and intends to identify, support, and train individuals in rural populations. This approach pre-empts incapacity, morbidity, and mortality, and at the same time enhances the probability of a functional community through retention in life-long motivation programmes.

ATC, a concept of service delivery in which all services are delegated to the community level (see Internal document NMT-HAART proposal to Stichting Liberty, 2002; see for definition also Wallace, 2002), provides comprehensive community health services, including quality primary health care, chronic disease management, reproductive health and support services like radiology and laboratory services. ATC is a community-based centre of excellence for integrated primary health, TB and HIV/AIDS care.

CHAMP, on the other hand, provides a society (individuals, families and the community at large) with a future orientation, through social transformation and individual achievement. CHAMP develops, motivates, and retains clients in support programmes through talent and skill development in music, sport, and further education.

RAP is based on the premise that all inhabitants in an underserved rural area are deprived of certain basic needs preventing them from leading a normal life and achieving realistic developmental goals. Contributing factors to the abnormality of isolated communities include poverty and its associated societal ills and implications. RAP believes that despite the deprivation, these communities possess a wealth of abilities, skills, talents, and networks that can be developed to achieve progress.

Figure 2 illustrates the progress of HIV over time, from HIV- to HIV+, from in-fected (but not affected) towards compromised disease that requires medical inter-vention and adherence management. Currently, most global HIV efforts and funding address the 'care & treatment' block in which infected patients are clinically treated for opportunistic infections and AIDS. The NCG view is that we try to:

- stop the massive number of sero-conversions through effective, evidence-based, community intervention programmes with the aim of behavioural change (pri-mary prevention);
- actively work on a generalised prevention programme: 'know your status, know your stage' campaign that promotes annual testing for the whole community, to detect HIV infection at an early stage (secondary prevention);
- actively work on early enrolment to control disease progress and initiate ARV treatment at an early stage (tertiary prevention);
- actively work on therapy adherence and community understanding of the disease profile (motivation).

If turning the tide of HIV and AIDS is unattainable, it would be impossible to elim-inate the backlog that increases daily. This means in practice reducing the number of full-blown AIDS patients on waiting lists, initiating ARV management earlier and achieving a non-acceptance of morbidity and mortality caused by HIV infection through this shift.

As the HIV epidemic attracts more attention, finances and resources than any other disease, RAP restructured its chronic disease management (diabetes mellitus, hyper-tension, cardiovascular diseases, etc.) and community development on the back of the HIV investment, by following the same continuum of care described above. The RAP approach towards managing HIV, with its emphasis on prevention and motiva-tion and with rural advancement as its outcome, is an appropriate strategy to reduce the rise in orphans, loss of employment, and economic decline in rural settings as it pre-empts breakdown. Figure 2 illustrates the opportunities that exist to prevent the progress of compromised chronic disease and poverty through prevention (aware-ness, screening, and staging) and the treatment and retention of subjects in pro-grammes. Prevention is any activity that reduces the burden of mortality or morbid-ity of disease, at any level.

This approach pre-empts and avoids the acute and expensive compromised phases of chronic illness and poverty, and proactively manages all the events through pre-vention (social marketing that leads to responsible behaviour, early detection, sta-ging), early intervention and adherence support across an individual's lifespan. The objective is to circumvent the morbidity and mortality stage altogether through effec-tive prevention, i.e. to straighten the time line. Once the time line is straightened, one can introduce motivation and growth opportunities to improve the community through the identification, grading and nurturing of talents, abilities, and skills in the population. NCG developed customised programmes to address each stage and age of life to ensure that an earlier investment in an individual is not neutralised by a care gap later on in life, e.g. an effective Prevention of Mother-to-Child Transmission

(PMTCT) programme only has value if the child is protected against HIV infection and malnourishment throughout his/her life.

In an attempt to work cost effectively and create job and career opportunities through the HIV investment, we attempt to develop local skills and employ people from the community, without compromising service quality. NCG follows a policy of delegation of tasks (and associated training) to the lowest level (rank) that can fulfil the task, and thereby builds capacity in the local community to sustain and improve both the programme and the community (task shifting).

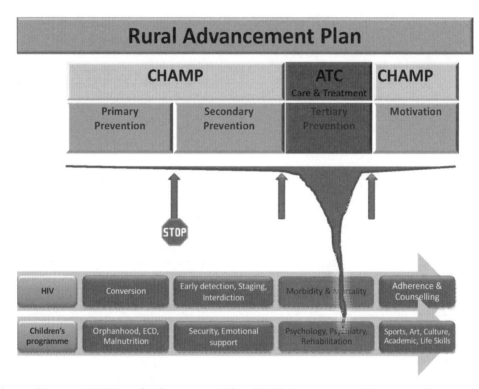

Figure 2: NCG Rural Advancement Plan (RAP): Autonomous Treatment Centre (ATC) & Community Care Health Awareness Mobilisation & Prevention (CHAMP) programme

In Figure 2, we visualise HIV as a time line starting with being HIV-. This stage represents primary prevention, and its objective is to prevent HIV- people from turning HIV+, represented by the Stop sign in the figure. If you turn HIV+ (sero-convert), you enter secondary prevention: you are now HIV+ but not yet affected or ill; this period usually lasts three to seven years. The objective of secondary prevention is early detection and early care-seeking behaviour to ensure good health through pro-active monitoring (CD4 and TB screening) and screening for opportunistic infections and symptoms of disease progress. When the CD4 count drops, then the line starts to decline. If ART is introduced early (CD4 350 or above), then de-compensation is averted, and clients can continue leading a normal productive life. This prevents people losing employment, falling seriously ill or dying. If clients are not initiated on ART at this stage, however, they start on the slippery slope towards full-blown AIDS. Through the intervention with ARV and rehabilitation, we can reverse this decline with long-term outcomes, for compliant patients, equal to the quality of life of HIV-people. However, this stage (tertiary prevention) requires professionally trained staff, drugs and often hospitalisation, resources that are expensive and often outside the reach of rural settings, and should be avoided to render the RAP effective. The next step in the continuum is to ensure the adherence of patients to lifelong treatment. Clients are motivated to comply with treatment regimens through support groups, follow-up visits, and skills development programmes.

In the figure, each time block has its own intervention programmes based on primary, secondary and tertiary prevention principles. Only the block of 'ATC Care & Treatment' requires qualified health care professionals (doctors, pharmacists, professional nurses, etc.). NCG trains local resources to deliver the rest of the continuum of care, under the supervision of the professionals. NCG also supports technologically advanced infrastructure and equipment to facilitate decentralisation and autonomy of the programmes. These centres of excellence attract professional skills to rural areas and motivate local inhabitants who qualify professionally to return to the rural community after graduating, supporting the scaling up of skills in these areas.

The CHAMP blocks reflect the services that trained counsellors and auxiliary health workers can supply if disease is detected early (VCT+), staged, and managed through effective maintenance and adherence programmes.

A central part of CHAMP concerns primary and secondary prevention intervention programmes. VCT+ is a major element and the entry point into the NCG strategy. In a country like South Africa, with a severe epidemic where around 30% of the adult population is HIV+, everybody is potentially affected, and everybody should know their status and stage of disease. VCT+ refers to counselling and testing that is immediately followed up by a CD4 count, to stage positive individuals at the time of testing, TB questionnaire screening, and staging to present these clients with an individual referral, treatment care and adherence plan. This practice improves patient adherence, compliance and retention in RAP programmes. NCG therefore achieves considerable economies of scale, skills development, and accesses a large numbers of clients in a cost-effective way.

NCG plans to replicate the RAP model in five sites by 2012 (see Figure 3):
1. NCG Ndlovu: Both the ATC model and CHAMP programmes are rolled out;
2. NCG Bhubezi: the ATC model and prevention programmes are implemented;
3. NCG Nyathi : under construction, planned opening first quarter of 2010;
4. NCG Bhejane: functions as a satellite of NCG Ndlovu, ATC opening: end of 2010;
5. NCG Ingwe: planned opening end of 2011.

Through NCG head office, Ndlovu creates and supports decentralised facilities that provide care to the different communities. NCG wants to operate five RAP sites by 2012.

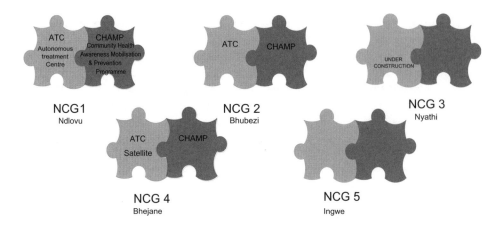

Figure 3: NCG RAP implementation programme

4.1. NCG Ndlovu

This RAP site is located in the Moutse valley, Limpopo, and serves a population of 120,000-140,000 people. NCG Ndlovu developed the model and formulated the RAP through trial and error over the years. There is no other medical or essential service infrastructure available in the valley, and about 40% - 70% of the residents are unemployed. At NCG Ndlovu, the NCG model is fully functional: community health services and community care services.

4.2. NCG Bhubezi

This NCG is located in Bushbuckridge, Limpopo, and serves a population of 70,000 people living in a radius of 50 km. NCG Bhubezi started in April 2007, and the community health services and community prevention programmes are currently operational. The rest of the services will be implemented as funding becomes available.

4.3. NCG Nyathi

NCG Nyathi, in the Utah district in Mpumalanga, will be the third site, and construction was completed in July 2009. The site is expected to open in 2010 in full partnership with the Department of Health and the initial donor Buffelshoek Trust.

4.4. NCG Bhejane

NCG supports the Waterberg Welfare Society (WWS), an NGO that has been active in the area of Vaalwater for more than ten years, as a satellite site. The site runs CHAMP and a HAART programme, and with appropriate investment, NCG wants to develop this as the fourth RAP.

4.5. NCG Ingwe

This site has not been identified and is only programmed for 2011.

Apart from these locations, NCG Ndlovu established a mobile team (nurses, counsellors, and administrative staff) to provide occupational HIV care on farms and in the workplace (the Farm project) and manages a for-profit Corporate Workplace Wellness Programme.

NCG's main aim is to integrate all of the programmes and strategies with the public sector programmes. NCG Ndlovu's ATC received full accreditation from DoH in July 2009, NCG Bhubezi received accreditation in October 2009, while NCG Nyathi and NCG Bhejane are busy with negotiations.

5. RAP Autonomous Treatment Centre (ATC)

Through the ATC, the RAP contributes to the following MDGs:
- Promote gender equality & empower women
- Reduce child mortality
- Improve maternal health
- Combat HIV/AIDS, malaria, etc.

ATC provides holistic community health services, with an emphasis on integrated quality primary health care, chronic disease management, reproductive health and support services. It is a community-based centre of excellence for primary healthcare, TB and HIV/AIDS care. As such, it addresses three of South Africa's major problems, namely:
- remigration of skills to rural areas;
- the creation of capacity and employment through comprehensive health delivery; and
- targeting HIV/AIDS and TB by providing care where the epidemic is at its worst: the rural areas.

The ATC programme consists of:
- a 12-hour Community Health Centre,
- a 24-hour Maternity and In-patient Clinic, and
- support and diagnostic services.

6. RAP Community Health Awareness Mobilisation and Prevention Programme (CHAMP)

Through the CHAMP, the RAP contributes to the following MDGs:
- Eradicate extreme poverty & hunger
- Achieve universal primary education
- Promote gender equality & empower women
- Combat HIV/AIDS, malaria, etc.
- Ensure environmental sustainability

CHAMP represents all community care programmes in the NCG portfolio, and although community health and community care operate as separate programmes, the success of RAP depends heavily on the quality of referrals amongst the programmes. CHAMP consists of the following programmes:

- Prevention programme;
- Children's programme;
- Sports, arts & culture programme;
- Community development programme;
- Community liaison.

7. Thoughts about a NCG Assessment and Change Concept

Behavioural change, improved quality of life and community development as the main outcomes of RAP require clear strategies, standardization, and priorities for implementation in new sites.

The first step in planning a new project or programme demands a thorough scan of the external environment, i.e. a needs analysis of the community in terms of demographic, political, economic, social, epidemiological and infrastructural or technological aspects. In line with ABCD principles, community assets fall into five categories: individuals, local associations, local institutions, physical assets and the local economy (including local business assets and local expenditures). After the environmental scan, the ABCD scan is the next step in determining community needs and community assets; this neighbourhood inventory forms the basis of the action plan. Priorities can now be set on the basis of a proven frame of reference. RAP utilizes Abraham Maslow's hierarchy of needs theory to prioritise community interventions. Maslow published the theory in 1954, and it remains valid today for understanding human motivation, management training, and personal development. It orders the five levels of human needs that Maslow identified: (1) physiological, (2) safety & security, (3) sense of belonging, (4) esteem, and (5) self-actualisation into a sequence or hierarchy. In terms of the theory, a lower order need must be fulfilled before the next level of need can be addressed. Unless the lower order needs are fulfilled, it is very difficult to motivate an individual towards achievement. RAP addresses the lower order needs through the CHAMP community involvement programmes and ATC programmes, while the higher order needs are addressed by the CHAMP sport, arts & culture, and children's programmes. In other words, the implementation of a RAP programme follows the needs analysis; programme design is determined by and adapted to the community's needs, rather than forcing the implementation of standardized programmes that do not fit the community agenda. The Maslow theory provides NCG with proven ecological validity and with a rationale for the attainment of the different NCG programmes that make up the RAP.

The next programmatic issue concerns the question of 'how' a programme is to be implemented and carried out. This means that communal assessment approaches and intervention strategies have to be developed. Communal assessment approaches involve a single strategy to include people in a needs analysis and the development and use of a set of assessment tools that fit each human need category. To this end, already existing assessment methods and instruments could be used. However, it will often be the case that these methods and instruments are not yet validated for the specific target population when they are developed in another country or in another socio-cultural setting. The user has to be aware that they could result in social-culturally biased outcomes. Another aspect of 'how to implement a programme' depends on the behaviour and community change strategy to be used. Many of the ones used by NGOs were developed or derived from strategies developed elsewhere. This implies that they could be culturally biased. NCG already has a lot of experience in the implementation of change strategies; and always attempts to establish support for the NCG programmes through evidence-based research. However, before such research can be started, it has to be clear what kind of philosophy or theory underpins the intervention strategy. After all, the purpose of a philosophy or theory is that it explains why a certain intervention could be expected to have specific outcomes. An example of such a theoretical starting point is the Theory of Planned Behaviour of Ajzen (1991), which provides a useful explanatory frame of reference for behaviour change.

To give the NCG programmes a well-considered common foundation, the Herzberg Two-Factor Theory and the AIDA Model for Buying Behaviour are utilised as a heuristic frame of reference. NCG wants to transfer, apply and test the Herzberg motivation-hygiene theory, a popular but controversial theory of employee satisfaction in the workplace, to social mobilisation. The two-factor theory unpacks the needs of individuals based on the Maslow hierarchy of needs and categorises them in terms of absent needs (hygiene) and motivational needs (motivators). The Herzberg theory relates these needs and their presence or absence to happiness (satisfaction with life). Consistent with the motivation-hygiene theory, positive psychologists are showing that happiness is more than the absence of unhappiness (Aspinwall & Staudinger, 2003; Seligman & Csikszentmihalyi, 2000). Motivator factors are essential to intrinsic motivation (Csikszentmihalyi, 1975; Deci, 1971; Deci & Ryan, 1985, 1991), and if these needs are addressed, then people learn, develop, and achieve their potential in life, and this increases their level of happiness. Hygiene factors contribute more to life dissatisfaction than to life satisfaction, and if these low-order needs are not satisfied, people are dissatisfied with life and consequently unhappy (Kahneman, Diener, & Schwarz, 1999; Kasser, 2002; Myers & Diener, 1996).

NCG wants to demonstrate how a two-step approach of identifying and addressing absent needs in the community and developing talents already present in the community can support positive ways of living and people's sense of a valued self-actualisation. We suggest that by drawing on theories and research from areas like psychology, sociology, health studies, and anthropology, it should be possible to devise risk-reducing and happiness-promoting behavioural change. The results from this can help to develop a set of guidelines or heuristics for the design of a social marketing campaign to effect behavioural change in the communities. For this purpose, NCG wants to transfer and test the AIDA model of buying behaviour as a social marketing strategy in rural settings. We would like to apply the principles of the AIDA model to the integrated model for behavioural change, to test whether an advertising strategy for consumer goods applies to selling prevention messages that lead to behavioural change outcomes. The AIDA model differentiates four stages in the buying process: (1) awareness, (2) interest, (3) decision and (4) action. The results from this study, if positive, could support a shift in emphasis from generic HIV & AIDS awareness (conventional prevention campaigns) towards a development programme and services that enhance well-being and promote less risky behaviour in a community.

To conclude, an important task for the future of NCG management and staff is the development of a common assessment and behaviour and community change concept.

8. NCG Management Structure

NCG has adopted a franchise model for the implementation of RAP that creates standardised policies and controls at a central level but leaves the accountability for implementation in the hands of those responsible for local outputs and outcomes. In this manner, it creates ownership at the local level while the head office evaluates and sets the standards. The NCG head office coordinates and controls all activities taking place at the NCG local level, but the local management enjoys a certain freedom to adapt the model based on community participation and feedback. The head office is also responsible for the planning, fundraising, development, and implementation of new NCGs.

The NCG head office supplies the support functions like human resource management, financial control, centralised fundraising, marketing, PR and branding, IT and IT development, centralised pharmacy procurement and standardisation of pharmacies to the local sites. Similarly, M&E and research are coordinated from the centre but implemented and executed at the local level.

NCG head office has an Executive Committee, led by the CEO, who reports to the NCG Board of Trustees. The CEO is responsible towards the Board of Trustees. The CEO manages NCG and is responsible for the overall achievement of NCG goals and objectives. The centralised NCG management and support team headed by the COO implements the strategy and ensures that all local programmes are standardised and that all programmes achieve efficiencies and quality outcomes.

NCG currently has around 240 full-time employees, of whom all but the specialists and professionals are recruited, trained, and promoted from the local community. NCG focuses on employment and skills development in local communities to deliver comprehensive community services to achieve its vision. The Royal Netherlands Embassy shares this vision and funds the NCG head office expert management team that supports all operations.

NCG has achieved many goals and objectives since 1994 and has been recognised nationally and internationally with a variety of prestigious awards.

The Board of Trustees consists of eight Trustees and the CEO. The trustees are persons who are all experts in their own field of interest. Their varied skills and background ensure that this board has a broad scope to serve the interests of NCG through coaching the CEO and the Executive Committee. Their backgrounds vary from corporate management to academics, national and international law and representation from the NGO world.

8.1. NCG Research Consortium

The Ndlovu Research Consortium (NRC) is an initiative of the Ndlovu Care Group (NCG). NCG acts as the head office and secretary of NRC, while NRC looks after the academic interests of NCG through:
- initiating research related to the NCG intervention programmes;
- documenting NCG achievements;
- scientifically underpinning new efforts;
- researching innovative ideas regarding community care and health intervention programmes.

Currently, the NRC has four partners:
- University of Pretoria, South Africa: Faculty of Medicine, Faculty of Public Health, and Faculty of Economics and Business Science;
- Utrecht University, the Netherlands: Faculty of Medicine, and Faculty of Social and Behavioural Sciences;
- UNISA, South Africa: Bureau of Market Research;
- Ndlovu Care Group, South Africa.

Ndlovu Research Consortium will further expand research collaboration with Utrecht University, UNISA and the University of Pretoria, to be executed by post-graduate as well as master students of the participating faculties of both universities. NRC will develop from this relationship and professionalize the care provided by NCG. The consortium consists of multidisciplinary international cooperation between universities and an NGO, aiming at improving community health and care in rural South Africa. The consortium provides structured cooperation, in particular by means of combined appointments of academic personnel in a participating university as well as the NCG. All participating organizations contribute in kind to the consortium. This cooperation is established through a signed contract between the participating organizations. The consortium strives for further cooperation with other universities and NGOs in the future.

Research questions originate from identified problems in the rural community and health care, and the participating universities provide teaching and research facilities for NCG personnel. NCG, in turn, provides possibilities for a practical or research term for students and staff of the participating universities. Relevant databases of the participating organizations are at each others' disposal after an agreed contract about whom, when and why a specific database will be used. The consortium will appoint a research coordinator who is located at NCG.

All reports, papers, articles, etc. to be published as a result of the efforts of the consortium have to meet internationally accepted scientific standards, and the same goes for subsidy requests on behalf of the consortium.

Research ideas from both universities as well as NCG will be compiled into collaborative research proposals that aim at:
- improving the care for the patients,
- improving community care,
- supplying research material for tertiary education,

– strengthening research capabilities.

Intellectual property will be established for each project individually. The NRC will actively seek grants for research funding and collaborations with other research institutes. NRC will act as a channel to attract clinical trials of new drugs or diagnostics which will be conducted, implemented and evaluated at the most appropriate NCG sites. Cohort data collected over the years will be accumulated and evaluated for research proposals. NRC will ultimately investigate the possibility to participate in commercial clinical trials in order to create financial stability and sustainability within the consortium.

8.2. Human Resource Management

As any organisation expands and grows in terms of funding, operations, workforce, numbers of branches and geographical spread, structural changes become inevitable, and human resource management (HR) needs increase. Working in isolated rural areas compounds the problem of recruitment, selection, and retention. In line with RAP, HR recruits and trains wherever possible from the local community. Vacancies are always advertised internally first to maximise local skills development. Talented local candidates are encouraged through bursaries and in-house training programmes to improve their skills and advance their careers.

The RAP strategy decentralises world-class infrastructure to rural areas and supports these operations with ongoing research. This attracts top candidates to these areas without compromising academic or technological progress. It also encourages the re-migration back to their communities of trained inhabitants who grew up in these areas.

The NCG recruitment strategy includes intensive advertising and screening processes to ensure that we attract candidates who fit the personality of NCG and select NCG as their employer of choice. Extensive marketing and national and international recognition of NCG as an innovator highlight our profile as a company of choice. We also embark on proactive headhunting for key positions through networking with similar organisations in the industry. NCG prides itself on its mentoring support and skills development practices. NCG refrains from recruiting from the government as this negates efforts to support government capacity building. NCG offers competitive remuneration packages that are benchmarked against industry and public service salaries.

8.3. IT Management

The real need of IT development covers integrated data collection, exchange, and processing for all our programmes. Through Anglo Coal, a corporate partner of NCG, the Health Source software offers a solution for integrated data management for NCG. This programme is user friendly, and provides an IT solution for primary health care, TB care and an ARV roll out site and also integrates it with ICD10 coding, pharmacy, laboratory, inpatient care, finances, billing for medical scheme claims, down referral to clinics, and even community intervention programmes like Community VCTs, etc.

The parties involved produce a Health Information System that is multi-disease orientated, has a full integration of services, and provides mobility to the patient. The aim is to adapt this programme to NCG needs and add modules for the CHAMP programmes. Also, the intention is to bring this programme to the NGO environment at no cost for the user other than the licenses needed for its functionality. The ultimate aim is to introduce this system to the public sector as an Integrated Care Information System for implementation all over South Africa.

8.4. Marketing and PR Strategy

NCG is the corporate brand for all external activities and communication. The advantages of one brand are:
- it is easier to understand for outsiders;
- all employees realise that they are working for the same group;
- all advertisements have only one logo;
- it guarantees a standard of care for the donor, the user and the observer if a programme/product is endorsed with the brand;
- individual locations and programmes are sub-branded;
- NCG communicates with various target groups, and appropriate communication is essential to satisfy all groups.

8.5. Financial Management

NCG will remain dependent on donor funding. The donor diversity of NCG is an important factor for financial stability, so that the risks are spread over a variety of donor profiles. Although it is our aim to create sustainability and less donor dependency through integration in the public domain, donor support will remain an integral part of the model as we have chosen to work in communities which are deprived of the most elementary services. This situation will not change in the near future given the current environment and shortage of investments in those areas.

The donor profile varies from institutional donors (PEPFAR/USAID, UNICEF, Royal Netherlands Embassy), to corporate donors (Virgin Unite, Anglo American, Vodacom, etc.), to target-specific donor organisations (Right to Care, Stichting Liberty, Nelson Mandela Children's Fund, etc.), to Ndlovu-specific donor organisations (Elandsdoorn Foundation, Tjommie Foundation and Tempelman Stiftung), and to individuals donating with specific aims within the projects and programmes.

Good financial governance and financial transparency are pre-conditions for future funding. NCG has a Financial Department with a Senior Financial Manager for policy-making and planning at the central level and operational staff departments at each local NCG RAP site.

9. NCG Strategy for the Coming Three Years (2010-2012)

With the establishment of NCG head office in 2008, a professional management team was appointed to facilitate the expansion described and to implement the NCG model and strategy.

The NCG wants to play a leading role in assisting the Department of Health and other relevant Departments improving the Districts Health Service delivery in rural South Africa. This will be achieved through strategic public private partnerships (PPPs) with the relevant government departments, institutional donors, corporate institutions, and private investors whereby NCG's role will be to coordinate these efforts and provide the management support. Through the implementation of ATC's the trust and confidence of the community will be restored in local service delivery and subsequently the CHAMP programmes will be rolled out as well.

NCG also wants to set standards and share a model to achieve rural advancement through clinical and community services that empowers these communities to take responsibility for social transformation in underserved areas. The aim of the assistance is Asset-Based Community Development. We have to utilise the assets present in the community, develop and educate those and employ and retain them in our care systems.

References

Aspinwall, L.G. & Staudinger, U.M. (Eds.). (2003). *A psychology of human strengths: Fundamental questions and future directions for a positive psychology.* Washington, DC: APA Books.

Csikszentmihalyi, M (1975). *Beyond boredom and anxiety.* San Francisco: Jossey-Bass Publishers.

Deci, E.L. (1975). *Intrinsic motivation.* New York: Plenum.

Deci, E.L. & Ryan, R.M. (1985). *Intrinsic motivation and self-determination in human behavior.* New York: Plenum Press

Deci, E.L. & Ryan, R.M. (1991). *Intrinsic motivation and self-determination in human behavior.* In: Steers, R.M. & Porter, L.W. (Eds.). *Motivation and Work Behavior, 5th Edition (pp. 44-58).* New York: McGraw-Hill, Inc.

Sachs, J.D. (2005). *The End of Poverty.* London: Penguin Books.

Seligman, M.E.P. & Csikszenmihalyi, M. (2000). Positive psychology: An introduction. *American Psychologist, 55,* 5-14.

South African National HIV Prevalence, Incidence, Behaviour and Communication Survey 2008.

Wallace, R.B. (2002). *Gale Encyclopedia of Public Health.* New York: The Gale Group Inc., Macmillan Reference.

WHO (2006).*Monitoring and Evaluation toolkit HIV, AIDS, Tuberculosis and Malaria. Second Edition.* Geneva: WHO

Chapter 2

The NCG Management Structure: Scaling the Rural Advancement Plan (RAP) Model through Community Franchising

Mariette Slabbert[a], Hugo Tempelman[b,c]

"One of the vices of the virtue of decentralisation is that people don't share ideas."
Dorothy Nevill (British writer 1826-1913)

Abstract

NCG uses a franchise model to deliver services to rural populations through the Rural Advancement Plan (RAP). NCG wants to transfer its community franchise model to other non-profit organisations and the government as a solution for social mobilisation. This form of franchising supports other NGOs that have viable, yet non-scalable programmes through replication and central support. Hence, the RAP community franchise model enhances scalability and social value creation through replication. These NGOs and the government can utilise the model, methodology and ongoing technical support from NCG. Rural illness has the pervasive distinction of increasing the vulnerabilities of individuals already living below the poverty line. In some ways, falling sick in rural families could equate to death because of isolation and the absence of appropriate facilities and diagnostic services. The RAP model strives to replicate its social and technological platform, tackling preventive health and delivering relevant and affordable, decentralised services to rural areas. NCG shares the South African (SA) national government vision and goals, including the Millennium Development Goals (MDGs), for rural health care in SA that state that District Health Systems services will (1) be as equal in quality and accessibility to rural people as urban services are to their clients; (2) be comprehensive; (3) have efficient referral systems; (4) fully involve local communities. This NCG community franchise model creates autonomous operations in targeted areas that are standardised, measured, and controlled through a central head office.

---

a. COO Ndlovu Care Group, Groblersdal, South Africa
b. CEO Ndlovu Care Group, Groblersdal, South Africa
c. Visiting Professor, Faculty of Social and Behavioural Sciences, Faculty of Medicine, Utrecht University, The Netherlands

1. Introduction

The WHO study, '*Decentralisation in healthcare, strategies and outcomes*' (Saltman, Bankauskaite & Vrangbaek, 2007), states the following: "The logic of decentralisation is based on an intrinsically powerful idea. It is, simply stated, that smaller organisations, properly structured and steered, are inherently more agile and accountable than are larger organisations."

"We underline the important role of local authorities in contributing to the achievement of the internationally agreed development goals, including the Millennium Development Goals"[1] (p. 39), Anna Tibaijuka, under-secretary general of the United Nations stated in the foreword to the 'Localising the MDGs' report'[2]: "It is important to realize this: even though the MDGs are global, they can most effectively be achieved through action at the local level. It is at the local level that inequalities between people (in a city) can be addressed. It is at the local level that safe drinking water, electricity and other services including health and education are provided, that garbage is collected and that food is sold at markets. In each city and town, there will be a local reality to be taken into consideration, and indeed the MDGs should be adapted to meet this reality. This is also the only way to make the most of local social capital and get the community involved" (New York, 1 Nov 2005).

The WHO report on the decentralisation of health systems and its management in Nepal[3] states that decentralisation is the most powerful driving force in improving the efficiency of health system performance and equity, narrowing the unmet demands of the community and its empowerment. The report explains further that it is essential to define the task to be decentralised and the roles and functions of the management system, establishing appropriate laws and enforcement, properly and in a stratified manner. Concurrently, the authority and responsibility need to be clearly defined and respected by all levels, and the process of de-concentration, delegation and devolution should be appropriately addressed in the context of the respective community. This report suggests the following strategic actions for effective district health systems:

1. Strong and sustained political commitment is needed to delegate authority and stop encroaching on authority already delegated.
2. The capacity of local bodies needs to be appraised, and they must be provided with the necessary training programmes so that all their actions are based on informed decisions.
3. The new role of various levels of central authorities should also be re-defined and restructured accordingly so as to avoid ambiguities in the discharging of functions.
4. Strengthen the process development: development of strategies, standards, norms and performance indicators.
5. District health systems management needs to be strengthened. Structured training programmes in a team-building approach should be conducted in the respective districts.
6. There is still no adequate analytical framework for systematically studying the achievement attained through the assessment of performance-based health outcomes for both preventive and curative components.

7. A task force should be established involving all stakeholders engaged in the process monitoring of utility-based research on the district health system, introducing new innovative choices for better health care performance in a district.
8. Widen the decision space for the local bodies.

In a country like South Africa, where around 80% of the community is still HIV-negative, NCG believes that not enough effort is directed towards measurable and evidence-based prevention programmes at the local level. The donor dollar has up to now mostly been invested in treatment programmes that address the crisis of rampant HIV and AIDS mortality and morbidity, but largely ignoring the entry of new cases that require treatment. If prevention aspects are ignored, people are left to their own discretion of when to access care. This often happens only when the disease is advanced and the patients are seriously ill, often as a result of the stigma associated with the diagnosis of HIV. It is crucial that new infections are minimised, not only to preserve health but also to protect these already vulnerable populations.

According to a DFID report, 'HIV and AIDS In-depth' (2009),[4] there will continue to be new infections, but if our prevention efforts are successful, the new infections should occur at an increasingly lower rate. Nonetheless, these people will need to be treated. It is crucial that new infections are minimised. Currently, for every two people (initiated) on treatment in the world, five people are newly infected.

SA has limited resources, and to manage the epidemic effectively and efficiently without compromising the quality of outcomes, all efforts should be aimed at preventing more infections, early case finding, and preventing morbidity and mortality of compromised patients. In line with NCG's strategy of primary, secondary and tertiary prevention (see Chapter 1), NCG believes that efforts should be aimed at primary and secondary prevention to pre-empt de-compensation and the cost associated with it.

It follows that HIV needs to be understood as both an emergency for those without treatment and as a chronic condition for those with it. Developed and developing country governments and donors therefore need to make long-term plans (beyond 2015) for funding and deploying an adequate response. All stakeholders need to understand that the management of the HIV/AIDS epidemic is not a medical issue only. To manage HIV properly demands the ultimate integration of social and behavioural sciences and social and clinical medicine to develop fully integrated, evidence-based programmes around prevention, screening, staging, care and treatment, and, most importantly, retention strategies to support compliance to lifelong treatment.

The Treatment Time Bomb report[5] into long-term access to HIV medicines in the developing world confirms NCG's sentiments and cites the following recommendations to manage the epidemic successfully:
1. Key organisations purchasing HIV medicines, such as the Global Fund, UNITAID and PEPFAR, require assurances from donors that financial commitments will be secured for the longer term.
2. Advocates of universal access to HIV treatment, care, and support need to agree on a common message to drive and maintain progress beyond 2015.
3. Treatment is needed to save lives, but prevention is the only way to manage the epidemic in the long term. Each infection averted saves years of treatment costs.

Developing country governments, international NGOs, donors and others should work together urgently to develop best practice recommendations on prevention-to-treatment spending ratios.

4. UNAIDS should collect data on the extent of the use of CD4 tests, and donors should stand ready to fund the rollout of a cheap, easy-to-use CD4 test as it becomes available. This could dramatically improve survival rates for people with HIV.

This means that HIV and AIDS strategies should be redesigned with a longer-term focus in mind to render services that are both sustainable and cost-effective. Direct and indirect costs associated with tertiary prevention or programmes that focus on treatment only require resources that are scarce and expensive, specifically in rural areas. These scarce and expensive resources include:

- Human resources: compromised clients often require professional care including doctors, nurses, pharmacists, dieticians, social workers, occupational therapists and management staff.
- Physical resources:
  - hospitalisation: compromised patients require intensive care and monitoring
  - expensive medication;
  - diagnostic testing including pathology and radiology;
  - specialised referrals.
- Transport and travel costs.
- Social costs:
  - compromised patients have a higher mortality rate, and this increases the likelihood of children losing their parents, and families without income;
  - the increased morbidity associated with illnesses often results in unnecessary job losses and deepening of poverty.

The RAP targets specific rural communities, demarcates a target area, identifies the needs, and addresses the needs holistically. NCG developed standardised policies, procedures, monitoring & evaluation frameworks, and supportive research to create a community franchise model for consistent delivery in different rural areas. NCG has a centralised head office that supplies guidance and support services, and that guides implementation at local sites. Through the focus on prevention, NCG develops and trains human resources available in the community to manage the epidemic whereby the responsibility for addressing the epidemic is delegated back to the affected community. This goes hand in hand with skills development, empowerment, and job creation, which acts as a catalyst for community development.

The South African Franchising Association[6] has published a practical definition of a franchise which states that it is a grant by the franchisor to the franchisee, entitling the latter to the use of a complete business package containing all the elements necessary to establish a previously untrained person in the franchised business, to enable him or her to run it on an ongoing basis efficiently and profitably, according to guidelines supplied.

2. Target group

NCG identifies rural populations with limited or no access to basic services and delivers community health and community care programmes, in cooperation with government and the private sector. Target areas are selected and demarcated to ensure that interventions are measurable and that action plans are attainable. The Center for Disease Control (CDC) describes community mobilisation as a process that engages all sectors of the population in a community-wide effort to address a health, social, or environmental issue. CDC states that community mobilisation brings together policy-makers and opinion leaders, local, state, and federal governments, professional groups, religious groups, businesses, and individual community members. Community mobilisation empowers individuals and groups to take some kind of action to facilitate change. Part of the process includes mobilising necessary resources, disseminating information, generating support, and fostering cooperation across public and private sectors in the community. NCG believes that community mobilisation, through franchising, is the credible way to address the poverty and disease burdens in the different underserved communities. NCG operates NCG Ndlovu in Moutse (Limpopo), NCG Bhubezi in Bushbuck Ridge (Mpumalanga), and NCG Bhejane in cooperation with Waterberg Welfare Society in Vaalwater (Limpopo); and NCG Nyathi in Utah (Mpumalanga) is under development in cooperation with Buffelshoek Trust. None of these target communities has access to basic healthcare, piped water, sewerage, waste removal, or postal services, and unemployment figures are rampant.

NCG maximises the individual potential in talented residents to build capacity in these areas. This strategy is referred to as Asset-Based Community Development (ABCD), which mobilises and accesses all community structures in a targeted community to screen, stage, develop and nurture community assets utilising the skills and abilities that already exist. Given the strain on government resources in SA, it is unlikely that rural areas will be supplied with services soon. SA is furthermore hampered by severe skills shortages and lack of infrastructure to provide clinical services in rural areas. This is demonstrated in widespread implementation problems and variations in service quality at the local level.

NCG works closely with civil society organisations, faith-based organisations, traditional healers and government structures at the local, provincial and national levels and aligns all its programmes with national guidelines and the MDGs.

3. Aims

Operating in a rural environment requires an understanding of working within and learning from a close-knit community's psychology, expectations, and constraints in order to design services that are relevant, accessible, and equitable.

Health sector reform in developing countries, including the decentralisation of management and the provision of primary health care, is expected to produce changes in the pattern of health service delivery and improvements in the equity of provision (Franchising, 2008; Hayes, 2006).[7] NCG supplies both centralised and decentralised services to its operations to achieve autonomy and quality at the implementation level through the community franchise model for rural advancement. The following players are involved in the RAP model:

- Private sector investor to develop and fund the necessary infrastructure if this is not available in the target area. Infrastructure includes:
  - 12-hour unit to supply comprehensive primary care;
  - 24-hour unit for ante- and postnatal, prevention of mother-to-child transmission (PMTCT), obstetric, and inpatient care;
  - support services to make rural facilities autonomous in its operations;
  - administrative offices that include a training facility.
- Local NGOs, FBOs and CSOs.
- Government departments including Departments of Health, Social Welfare, Home Affairs, Justice, Arts & Culture, infrastructure development.
- NCG supplies the model and central management supports for effective implementation, monitoring and control. This includes certain local level appointments: senior manager of clinical care, senior manager of community care, monitoring and evaluation, community liaison, and financial expertise.

3.1. NCG Management

NCG has adopted a franchise model for the implementation of the RAP that creates standardised policies and controls at a central level but leaves the accountability for implementation in the hands of those responsible for local outputs and outcomes.

NCG Head Office supplies the support functions like human resource management, financial control, fundraising, marketing, public relations and branding, information technology (IT) and IT development, pharmacy procurement and standardisation of pharmacies to the local sites. These functions are coordinated from the centre but implemented, executed, and controlled at the local level.

3.2. Human Resource Department

Working in isolated rural areas compounds the problem of recruitment, selection, and retention. The HR department recruits and trains whenever possible from the local community.

The strategy of local skills and ability development requires intensive formal and on the job training but leads to the reward of local employment and resultant social mobilisation.

The HR department is responsible for the following outputs:

- Recruitment, selection, and induction;
- Conditions of employment and employee benefits in line with current legislation;
- Internal labour relations and employee relations;
- Performance management;
- Education and training;
- Management of the payroll.

Each of these functions has both a central and local dimension (see Table 1).

Table 1: Central and local dimensions of HR functions

Central	Local
Recruitment, Selection and Induction	
– Updating of recruitment policies and maintenance of best practices in recruitment and selection practices – Developing key industry partnerships to maximise recruitment efforts – Overseeing and controlling recruitment processes – Advertising, short listing and interviewing professional and management position candidates and negotiating job offers with potential candidates – Reporting to managers and the COO on recruitment and selection on a monthly basis – Ensuring that all positions have updated job profiles and that all recordkeeping is done – Immigration administration for foreign employees – Developing, leading, and managing the induction procedures in liaison with local management and local HR personnel – Ensuring follow-up through meetings, formal and informal discussions, and assisting new employees to settle positively and productively in new positions	– Placing of advertisements of vacancies and updating the spreadsheet of the candidate's profile for management short-listing for junior positions – Compiling CVs, questionnaires for the interviewers, contacting successful candidates to advise on the company's induction process, and reminding managers about the arrival of new appointees – Arranging hosts to provide tours of facilities and introduction to management, employees and other stakeholders – Collecting all documentation from new employees and explaining HR policies and procedures – Follow-ups (through meetings, discussions) formal and informal, assisting employees to settle positively and productively in new position – Maintaining employee personnel file
Conditions of Employment, including Remuneration Policy	

– Reviewing and updating conditions of employment according to applicable legislation i.e. Labour Relations Act (LRA), Basic Conditions of Employment Act (BCEA), Unemployment Insurance Fund (UIF) and Compensation for Occupational Injury on Duty Act (COIDA)
– Managing and coordinating remuneration policy, developing policies to cover key issues of conditions of employment, and checking that termination procedures are adhered to
– Reviewing and conducting of exit interviews and managing retrenchment of employees according to laid down statutory instruments
	– Implementing conditions of employment as per Acts
	– Leave administration, i.e. policy communication, enforcement and recordkeeping and administration of regulatory matters according to applicable legislation.
	  – Update UIF membership monthly and complete application forms for employees for unemployment claims
	  – Complete COIDA forms for any work-related injuries of employees and respond to any claim queries that may arise
	  – Keep employees informed about any changes, update records and ensure employees comply with the BCEA
	  – Ensure coordinators maintain attendance registers for all personnel

Employee Benefits (EB)	

– Ensuring that administration of employee benefits is updated monthly	– Informing service providers about staff movement and compensation on:
	  – Medical aid
	  – Provident Fund

Central	Local
– Signing off monthly employee benefits, reconciliation and negotiating with service providers on benefit structure – Communicating and educating management and employees on employee benefits through workshops, group meetings and individual discussions and managing benefit queries from management	– Group Life cover – Arranging communication and education of staff and employees on employee benefits through workshops, group meetings and individual discussions – Registering, documenting, recordkeeping and updating employees on benefits and unemployment – Managing benefit queries from management and employees

Internal Labour Relations and Employee Relations

Central	Local
– Designing, documenting and implementing disciplinary codes (processes and procedures) and outcomes, and ensuring that discipline in the company is according to the disciplinary code, and assisting management on implementation of the disciplinary code – Arbitrating and conciliating disciplinary code between employees and management – Informing staff representatives and management about labour law developments and amendments – Facilitating effective employee relations through diagnosing and solving complicated personnel problems – Liaising and negotiating with internal employee forum/union, regulatory bodies i.e. Department of Labour and CCMA where necessary – Liaising with labour relations organisations such as trade unions, CCMA with regard to industrial relations – Ensuring that processes and procedures are in place for industrial relations management	– Documenting and implementing disciplinary codes (processes and procedures) for staff (e.g. suspension, non-payment of salary as a disciplinary measure) – Enforcing rules and regulations as per the disciplinary code – Arbitrating and conciliating disciplinary code between employees and management – Informing staff representatives about labour law developments and amendments – Archiving of all disciplinary documents in employee files – Attending to and resolving staff welfare issues

Performance Management

Central	Local
– Developing, documenting and implementing performance management systems – Facilitating the transformation of the organisational culture towards a performance-driven culture through the implementation of performance management using the Balanced Scorecard – Managing and documenting the annual performance review process, ensuring adherence to agreed processes and procedures by both management and employees – Advising line managers on poor performance counselling and on managing key performers and overseeing implementation of poor performance counselling recommendations – Ensuring the completion of Performance Development Plans, setting up a talent manage-	– Informing managers of due dates, facilitating and documenting the annual performance review process, ensuring adherence to agreed processes and procedures by both management and employees – Advising line managers on poor performance counselling for general staff – Overseeing implementation of poor performance counselling recommendations and maintaining records of all performance management process flow – developmental plans, career plans, etc. – Recording training and education needs against project objectives and performance management outcomes and processing training needs for staff and liaising with finance department for payments

Central	Local
ment framework, and advising managers to develop Succession Plans – Managing key positions	– Keeping records of all training interventions for compilation of the annual training report to the Health and Welfare SETA

Management of Payroll

Central	Local
– Checking and approving Salary Spreadsheet for monthly payroll changes from HR Officers at the local level – Reviewing and signing off monthly payroll after processing on VIP – Reviewing and approving reconciliation of payroll creditors (SA Revenue Services (SARS), UIF, Medical Aid, Provident Fund, Group Life)	– Informing Salaries Administrator about changes to monthly payroll – Calculating overtime and reviewing monthly payroll after processing on Payroll – Advising Salaries Officer of payroll changes and advising service providers (medical scheme, Provident Fund and Group Life), documentation and related administration

3.3. NCG Information Technology

NCG tries to consolidate all its data collection in a single comprehensive data programme, the Health Source. The Health Source is a programme developed and made available to NCG by Anglo American, under its corporate social responsibility programme. The Health Source is an extensive Electronic Health Record for clinic, hospital and occupational health services with integrated functions for the pharmacy, laboratory, X-ray, stock control, costing and billing. At this stage NCG still has separate data systems for the Child Care and Community Care Programmes, but these modules are under development with Anglo support.

Due to the rural environment that the clinics operate in and the poor telecommunication infrastructure there, localised support is essential for the day-to-day operations of local sites. At the moment NCG relies on the use of privately owned wireless networks for data communications between the sites and service providers and is limited by what these service providers can offer. This implies that web-based programmes are difficult to implement, slow, and often frustrating for the user. Local servers mean no live data for central management, with the compromise of local servers and batch data transfer at night to central.

When new telecom networks become available, more services will be centralised. A more centralised approach would reduce infrastructure costs and simplify system maintenance. To run smooth communication networks among sites and head office, a major upgrade in the telecommunication infrastructure would be needed. Increased centralisation does not imply that local support would not be necessary as the sites all have large numbers of users that need desktop and other logistical support on site.

Centralised Services:
– Software development; development of new programmes;
– Company intranet/extranet to ensure connectivity;
– Custom application hosting;
– Remote server support;
– Security and policy control;
– Integration with financial systems.

Localised Support
- Local network administration functions;
- Desktop and end-user support for in-house operators;
- Pharmacy applications to support pharmacy management and dispensing software;
- Laboratory system integration with HealthSource;
- Radiology: digital imagery and sonar support.

The real need of IT development lies in integrated data collection, exchange, and processing for all our programmes. The Health Source software offers a solution for integrated data management. This programme is user-friendly and provides an IT solution not only for Primary Health Care, TB care and an ARV roll-out site, but integrates it with ICD10 coding, pharmacy, laboratory, inpatient care, finances, billing for medical scheme claims, down referral to clinics, and even community intervention programmes like community HCTs, etc.

The parties involved will produce a Health Information System that is multi-disease orientated, has full integration of services, and provides mobility to the patient. The aim is to adapt this programme to NCG needs and add modules for the CHAMP programmes. There is also the intention to bring this programme to the NGO environment at no cost to the user other than the licenses needed for its functionality. It is the ultimate aim to introduce this system to the public sector as an Integrated Care Information System for implementation all over South Africa.

3.4. Marketing and Communication

NCG established a corporate brand that represents and communicates all its operations. The local sites are sub-branded in line with the central brand and the corporate communications manual. Central marketing develops all marketing and communication materials and supplies the sites with the tools:

Central Marketing:
- The centralised marketing strategy controls the image of the group in line with the NCG values: fun, funky, holistic, dynamic, and innovative.
- The differences in sociological, geological and other environmental factors of the various locations influence the planning and controlling procedures used for marketing. Cultural aspects may differ for given communities, and therefore the marketing to individual communities is prepared in terms of the cultures served, and customized strategies communicate with the different communities.
- Customer relationship management for marketing to national and international donors, partners, and clients is centralised, and localized in terms of provincial and local authority and civil society organization networking. It is vital for NCG to retain the various external marketing and advertising campaigns for customer/donor/investor liaison under centralized control to guarantee consistent messaging.
- Customer relationship management with the relevant governmental partners is pivotal in our strategy to align and embed our programmes in the different Na-

tional Strategic Plans. Through our marketing and relationship building with the relevant government departments, the sustainability of our service delivery must become assured over time.

- NCG has developed a strong visual campaign (billboard, electronic media, and poster) that addresses issues bluntly to de-stigmatize and achieve behavioural change in clients; the group wants to integrate this campaign with national information and education campaigns that concentrate on awareness rather than behavioural change.
- Central marketing campaigns include a website, monthly digital newsletters, newspaper and magazine articles, radio interviews, publication of research articles, presentations at conferences and seminars, and personal selling to donors and government stakeholders.

Local Marketing:
- A community liaison officer at each site ensures that operations are aligned with the community's interests. These officers constantly feed information back to the central head office.
- NCG also allows for decentralisation through local site feedback from employees to compile marketing strategies, with the final approval authority maintained centrally.
- The CHAMP prevention programme delivers the social marketing messaging through a formally monitored and researched behavioural change communication campaign.

3.5. NCG Monitoring & Evaluation

Monitoring and Evaluation (M&E) is about discovering what actually works in providing a service, so that those receiving services are satisfied and those planning and delivering services can improve over time. NCG relies on evidence-based information to make programmes work and to channel financial resources accurately. This depends on functional monitoring and evaluation that are carried out at different levels in the organization. In the RAP model, the M&E function is managed centrally by an M&E manager who oversees all M&E-related functions and processes. At this level, the functionality of M&E is supported by other services such as IT, Learning and Development (L&D), Marketing and Communication, Epidemiology, the Ndlovu Research Consortium, and HR, as discussed in the chapter on M&E (chapter 4).

Human Resources

One of the requirements of the organization is that M&E functions are embedded in the job descriptions and performance agreements of all relevant staff.

Finance Department

The M&E reporting programme is linked to the in-house financial management systems. Project financial management is based on flows of information relating to implementation progress, income, expenditure, and other financial functions of the programmes. This is to enable both effective financial management and audit functions.

Central M&E Function and Localisation of M&E Processes

Central M&E ensures and institutes the development of an effective and efficient system for tracking the programmes, projects and activities that are ongoing in the local sites, and generates timely reports for the executive management and other stakeholders. This involves:

1. Preparing guidelines, training manuals and building M&E capacity on an ongoing basis:
   - Since monitoring involves collecting, analysing, and reporting data on inputs, activities, outputs, outcomes, impacts and external factors, there need to be guidelines on how the data are to be collected, analysed and reported. Central M&E thus ensures that there are systems and reporting templates in place to collect and analyse data, all of which are used by programme staff at the local sites (standardised systems and tools). Although the systems are centrally developed, the process is participatory and engages the local sites to give input and to ensure maximise benefits from the systems.
   - The M&E manager ensures that the capacity of local staff in terms of M&E tasks and processes is developed to ensure that the M&E coordination functions are localised in order to be effective in responding to day-to-day needs arising from community activities.
2. Ensuring that M&E is not carried out as an academic exercise, or a chore to satisfy donors, but that it is seen as a process leading to improved quality and coverage of services:
   - The benefits of having localized M&E functions are that this helps to increase participation by those people who benefit from the interventions and want to learn from the experiences of the programme. This is ensured by processes and M&E systems that ask the right questions for improving services and processes:
     - To what extent is M&E a set of participatory processes involving many stakeholders at local levels?
     - To what extent are data from monitoring shared between stakeholders?
     - To what extent are the experiences and views of service users captured in this process?
     - To what extent are future planning and service delivery based on lessons emerging from M&E?
   - NCG uses stakeholder platforms to jointly evaluate the results of monitoring and take action to address problems.

3.6. NCG Pharmaceutical Services

The Central Pharmacy Manager responsible for procurement at the central level ensures that the pharmacies adhere to good pharmacy practice (GPP):
- stock is available when and where needed;
- operations are cost-effective by capitalising on bulk purchases;

- there is efficient use of standard operating procedures
- waste is minimised, FIFO (First In First Out) procedures are implemented, expiry dates are checked, etc.;
- an appropriate infrastructure or 'quality system' encompassing the organisation structure, procedures, processes and resources exists;
- the systematic actions are in place for standardised 'quality' outcomes.

At the local level, the Central Pharmacy Manager has to ensure that there are procedures to monitor and maintain the quality of medicines from the moment they are received until they are consumed by the patient according to GPP guidelines:
- proper storage conditions and distribution procedures;
- appropriate pick and pack procedures;
- product defect reporting systems;
- adverse effect reporting systems;
- qualified personnel;
- quality assurance:
  - services are designed and developed correctly:
  - all operations are defined;
  - managerial responsibilities are defined in job descriptions;
  - checks are performed;
  - proper storage, distribution and handling of stock.

3.7. Financial Aspects of NCG

The Ndlovu Finance Department is divided into both a centralised and a decentralised function.

The central finance office provides the following services to the operations:
- Consolidation of financial and management reports
- Monitoring of internal controls
- Compilation of budgets and input into pre-award proposals
- Central banking and money market/treasury transactions
- Financial reports to donors
- Central payments
- Statutory activities and returns
- Company registration and secretarial functions
- Conducting and management of external and internal audits
- Central support services
- Central petty cash management
- Writing of finance policies and procedures, and job descriptions
- HR management in the finance office
- Asset management

The local functions of the finance department include:
- Local reconciliation and banking
- Local financial administration

- Petty cash management
- Implementation of internal controls
- Implementation of donor compliance
- Local level internal and external audits
- Transactional authority is vested in the local finance administrator and the clinic services manager
- Management reports
- Financial reports

3.8. NCG Local Operations

In order to manage local sites as autonomous units, NCG localizes several operational activities to maximize efficiencies; some examples include:
- Standardised continuum of care through primary, secondary, tertiary prevention and retention through motivation. This strategy prevents morbidity and mortality and retains clients in NCG programmes for life.
- Entry points into NCG programmes that include all ages and stages of life:
  - Ante- and postnatal care
  - PMTCT
  - Family medicine
  - In-hospital care
  - CHAMP children's programme:
    - Orphans & vulnerable children
    - Child-headed households
    - Nutritional units (malnourished children)
    - Pre-schools
    - Life skills training (school-going children)
    - Environmental education
  - CHAMP prevention programme:
    - Secondary schools programme
    - Community programmes
    - Civil society organisations
  - Community development programmes:
    - Entrepreneurial activities
    - Water programmes
    - Waste management
- Medical Waste Management: NCG developed decentralised incinerators that dispose of medical and other waste in a safe and effective way, in line with national and international safety standards. Needle incinerators in all cubicles minimise needle prick injuries.
- Technology: Advanced technology and digitalisation ensures interfacing and inter-referral amongst programmes:
  - Biometric scanning identifies clients that enter NCG programmes from different entry points.

- Decentralised laboratory can fully support the monitoring of HIV-positive clients on site. This ensures short turnaround times and minimises mistakes and loss of samples and specimens.
- Decentralised radiology services: digital x-ray facilities ensure high-quality imaging and easy referral to off-site second opinions. Digitalisation, although it has a high initial cost, is cost efficient in the longer term as it does not incur X-ray film and reagent costs; it decreases logistics management and optimises the results.

4. Conclusion

The NCG management model with shared central and local management services oversees and controls the quality and functionality of the model. This management model developed over time as a tool to facilitate local expansion.

Local baselines that consider cultural and/or environmental circumstances before starting new local sites ensure that the programmes fit their community environments from the outset. The fact that operations are supported by centralised specialist resources ensures that quality control is maintained, the local environment feels supported, and interactive reporting is ensured.

Standardization, with flexibility for customized local programmes, guarantees successful adoption of the franchise model in targeted communities. This model ensures that National Strategic Plans are implemented and that programmes report accordingly. The localized implementation of the MDGs integrates the government objectives to achieve these goals at the district and local levels.

The United Nations Report of the Global Forum on Innovative Policies and Practices in Local Governance[8] aptly states that while decentralization or decentralizing governance should not be seen as an end in itself, it can be a means for creating more open, responsive, and effective local government and for enhancing representational systems of community-level decision-making. It further states that by allowing local communities and regional entities to manage their own affairs, and through facilitating closer contact between central and local authorities, effective systems of local governance enable responses to the people's needs and priorities to be heard, thereby ensuring that government interventions meet a variety of social needs. The implementation of sustainable human development strategies will therefore increasingly require decentralized, local, participatory processes to identify and address priority objectives for poverty reduction, employment creation, gender equity, and environmental regeneration.

NCG is an NGO which is able to assist provincial and district authorities in this participatory process at a community level, supporting the relevant departments to strengthen the local service delivery and achieve their goals.

Notes

1. World Summit Outcome Document: United Nations, A/60/L.1*, 20th September 2005, para 173, page 39

2. Localising the Millennium development goals: a guide for municipalities and local partners, page iv
3. http://www.nep.searo.who.int/LinkFiles/Home_Dececentralisation_of_Health_System.pdf. WHO country Office, Nepal
4. DFID HIV and AIDS In-depth 2009; http://www.dfid.gov.uk/Global-Issues/How-we-fight-Poverty/HIVand AIDs/HIV-and-AIDS-in-depth
5. All-party Parliamentary group on AIDS, July 2009
6. http://www.bowman.co.za/IntellectualProperty/Franchising.asp
7. Senior Registrar in Public Health Medicine, Northern Region, Newcastle-upon-Tyne, England, on secondment to the Ministry of Health and Social Services, Windhoek, Namibia.
8. United Nations (DDSMS and UNDP), Report of the United Nations Global Forum on Innovative Policies and Practices in Local Governance, Gothenburg, Sweden, 23-27 September 1996, ref St/Tcd/Ser.E/46, p. 26

References

Franchising Etc. (2008). *Wat is franchising? Digitaal document (22 pp.).* Uitgever: Franching Etc..

Hayes, R (2006). *The Franchise Handbook: A complete Guide to All Aspects of Buying, Selling or Investing in a Franchise.* UK: Amzone.com

Saltman, R.B., Bankauskaite, V. & Vrangbaek, K. (eds.) (2007). *Decentralisation in healthcare: strategies and outcomes.* Berkshire, UK: McGraw-Hill.

WHO (1996). *Good Pharmacy Practice (GPP) in Community and Hospital Pharmacy Settings.* Geneva: World Health Organization.

Chapter 3

Cooperation and Alignment Amongst Stakeholders

Hugo Tempelman[a,b]*, Mariette Slabbert*[c]

> *"The Brave may not live forever, but the Cautious do not live at all."*
> Richard Branson (2009)

Abstract

This chapter first describes the combined task of the stakeholders towards creating sustainable solutions for South Africa. Stakeholders driving the process of social and economic development in rural areas include not only the government and the private commercial sector, but also the civil society organizations which are important change agents in the development of rural areas through their intimate understanding of the communities they operate in. Next, it describes the history of the national handling of the HIV epidemic and the antagonism amongst the stakeholders, with health care delivery as an example. Suggestions are made for the roles of each of the major stakeholders towards a sustainable synergetic solution for combatting the HIV and AIDS and TB epidemics in particular. Finally, the Ndlovu Care Group model for combined stakeholder participation in filling the treatment gap and poverty trap in the rural areas is outlined at the end of the chapter.

1. Introduction

After almost 15 years of the New South Africa, little has changed in most of the rural areas. Before 1994, the homelands were subjected to processes which can best be described as the development of underdevelopment; the challenge now is to amend these processes and implement sustainable activities that will reverse the 'trek from rural to urban'.

A considerable proportion of the South African population lives in poverty in the rural areas. Some 70% of the poor live in these areas. The non-urban population amounts to 45% of the total population, and of them 85% lives in the impoverished former homelands with unemployment rates exceeding 40-50%. Many other households have intimate ties to the rural areas through the migrant labour system.

There have been consistent government attempts to introduce modern services especially to the former homeland areas which have been particularly neglected and

---

a. CEO Ndlovu Care Group, Groblersdal, South Africa
b. Visiting Professor, Faculty of Social and Behavioural Sciences, Faculty of Medicine, Utrecht University, The Netherlands
c. COO Ndlovu Care Group, Groblersdal, South Africa

isolated, but these services are still very scattered, unreliable and out of reach for many who live in rural areas.

The national government chose to develop the rural areas in South Africa through the implementation of decentralized local governance structures. It is unfortunate for these areas that the development of local government was not a priority when this system was introduced; there is currently a lack of human resource capacity that hampers the implementation of the Integrated Sustainable Rural Development Strategy (ISRDP). Without deliberate local capacity building of the existing resources, this system will not gain momentum in self-governance to create the infrastructure needed to recruit and retain those individuals who are essential for sustainable service delivery in these disadvantaged areas; quality teachers, health professionals, programme management, entrepreneurial developers, etc.

Rural development should be seen from three important, independent but successive perspectives:
- social development;
- economic development;
- governance structures.

With reference to Chapter 1, these perspectives refer back to normalization of the circumstances through primary and secondary prevention and social development, including stable local governance, and only after a certain level of normalisation has taken place can one start to implement motivation and further upliftment through economic development. Social development, in turn, focuses on three important issues for advancing rural areas. These issues improve the capabilities of individuals, and they include, in this sequence:
1. infrastructure development that addresses physiological, safety, and security needs;
2. education to ensure that further education and training is an option for individuals; and
3. comprehensive healthcare that facilitates physical and mental development and productivity.

These three issues are key priorities for building local capacity, for retaining resources and achieving economic development. This will bring back the currency into the rural areas in the longer run, through which we increase local economic growth, decrease migrant labour and improve service delivery.

Economic development in impoverished rural areas where there is no currency available does not result in sustainable development because although there is a demand for products, there is no means to create a market system. It is therefore imperative that economic development follows social development in order to create a sustainable environment. It has to be a mix: the one cannot be envisaged or implemented without the other, but economic development without social development merely creates expectations and hope that is not sustainable. The sustainability becomes visible when the social development is followed by economic development that creates normalisation and incentives in the upscaled socio-economic environment. This is exactly what we mean by *"Retention through Motivation"* in our model (see Chapter 1 and 11).

Stakeholders driving the process of social and economic development include not only the government and the private commercial sector, but also the civil society organizations which are important change agents in the development of rural areas through their intimate understanding of the communities they operate in. Civil society organizations (CSO) or non-governmental organizations (NGO) bridge the gap between for-profit organisations and governmental service delivery and can be critical to effective delivery, both by assembling a clear inventory of people's needs and by fostering advocacy and cooperation in the implementation of improved delivery. A key constraint in rural development is an adequate civil society response. The CSO/NGO environment can be the catalyst between the needs/requests for services of a community and the public sector's response to deliver those services. Assistance in social development at a community level is the main task of the CSO/NGO fraternity.

Ndlovu Care Group utilizes asset-based community development (ABCD) principles to map the resources already available in rural areas and to utilize these civil structures as vehicles for buy-in and successful implementation.

2. The National Health Context of the Rural Areas

The rural areas of our country represent the worst concentrations of poverty. No progress can be made towards human dignity for our people as a whole unless we ensure the development of these areas. The government is now in a position to implement an integrated rural development programme. This will bring together all government departments and all spheres of government, including the traditional leaders. The integration we seek must ensure, for instance, that when a clinic is built, there is a road to access it. It must be electrified and supplied with water. It must have the requisite personnel, qualified to meet the health needs of the particular community. The safety and security of the personnel and the material resources which are part of the clinic must be guaranteed. We must also establish the conditions which enable this medical centre to radiate outwards as a point of reference with regard to the larger project of our self-definition as a people at work, building a better life for ourselves (Mbeki, 2002; p. 40). In order to make it worthwhile for people to remain in rural areas to provide the services, we have to economically develop the regions along with social development to create a sustainable environment.

Jocelyn Finlay (2007)[1] analyses the role of health in economic development via two channels: (1) the direct labour productivity effect and (2) the indirect incentive effect. The labour productivity hypothesis asserts that individuals who are healthier have higher returns on labour input. This has been well tested in the empirical literature with mixed conclusions. The incentive effect is borne of the theoretical literature: individuals who are healthier and have a longer life expectancy will have the incentive to invest in education as the time horizon over which returns can be earned is extended. Education is the driver of economic growth, and thus health plays an indirect role. Finlay concludes that without recognition of the indirect role of health, the economic benefits of health improvements are underestimated.

Piot (UNAIDS) stated in 2008 that there is a "need to revigorate the fight against the pandemic of HIV/AIDS by adopting a new response, namely to combine continuing crisis management and a long-term sustainable response" (p. 7).

The relevance of this remark is evident for South Africa as the epicentre of the global epidemic. The latest statistics reveal that at the end of 2007 about 5.7 million South Africans were living with the virus, with a prevalence level of 18%. Although the country has the biggest ARV roll-out response in the world, there is still a treatment gap of an equivalent size. Approximately one million South Africans have enrolled for treatment, and an equal number are in dire need of treatment but cannot access it due to a lack of capacity in service delivery. No access to service points, under-resourced and over-burdened clinics which cannot handle the needs of the community, lack of professional skills, etc. are all causes that contribute to the treatment gap. This problem is especially prominent in the rural areas. It is here where the major task of concurrent social and economic development has to take place.

Although the SA National HIV Prevalence, Incidence, Behaviour and Communication Survey 2008 suggests that the epidemic is stabilising and that the incidence may be declining, South Africa already has a high prevalence of HIV with a large infected pool. The ambitious target in the HIV and AIDS and STI Strategic Plan for South Africa 2007-2011 (NSP) of halving new infections reinforces the extent of the challenge posed by the epidemic and hence the need to scale up and intensify the national HIV response, regarding not only access to treatment and care, but especially evidence-based prevention and behavioural change programmes delivered in the communities, mobilising these communities to action at all levels. These are all issues which need to be addressed at a local level through the development of capacity and infrastructure. In order to achieve these aims, we have to ensure that the capacity we build or attract remains in those areas.

The impact of these challenges stretches far beyond the health sector to demographic, social and economic consequences for the country.

The complexity of what is described above leads to the question: "who is responsible for an adequate response?" The only remedy seems to be a comprehensive, long-term response that is guided by more partners and is a mix of social development and economic development, creating sustainable uplifting.

A well-known example of early economic development without the currency to sustain it is the Telkom example: Telkom achieved the rollout of 2.67 million new lines, mostly to poor households, within the 5-year period of its fixed-line exclusivity. However, only 667,039 of the new lines delivered were still in service by the end of that period.[3] It is argued that the bulk of the over 2 million cut-offs "were associated with increased household income poverty."[4] It proves the point that economic development before normalisation of certain aspects within a community does not automatically lead to sustained business or improvement of service delivery, despite the scope of the effort.

The provision of public health will always remain the responsibility of the government, mainly through the Department of Health, but unfortunately, the governmental resources (financial, infrastructural, material, human and logistic) are insufficient to address health care needs including the double epidemic of TB and HIV & AIDS.

The government, civil society organisations, business sector, corporate or SMEs and the private health care industry all share a responsibility towards health service delivery because it affects all of them. What is lacking at this stage is the appreciation of the responses given by the different stakeholders and of the effect that a combined response could have on the situation. Synergy amongst the stakeholders will eventually lead to a better understanding of each other and growth of mutual respect, whereby the relationship will develop towards partnership instead of working in isolation with diminished effect.

3. History

As an illustration of how the cooperation and coordination have failed between the different stakeholders that could have assisted with the Reconstruction and Development Plan for the rural areas, we can describe the history of the handling of the HIV epidemic.

The handling of the HIV/AIDS epidemic in South Africa has been dictated and directed by a political history that we cannot ignore when we discuss the subject of this chapter from the perspective of the Ndlovu Care Group. This history of a mismanaged emerging epidemic that turned political divided the parties. The same history delayed an adequate response when the epidemic was still controllable. The political decision to treat came before the political commitment was there. After the initial success of the mass roll-out of antiretroviral (ARV) programmes, we have to evaluate long-term sustainable solutions to map the way forward. In a country like South Africa, this can only be achieved through combined efforts and aligned strategies. It has to become a strategy of mass mobilisation of all layers of the population and government, including evidence-based prevention interventions combined with sustainable motivation programmes. This huge task can only be achieved if we combine the efforts of all major stakeholders. They include the South African government, especially the Department of Health, civil society organisations, specifically non-governmental organisations, and the business sector (corporate, SMEs) and institutional donors.

The initial implementation of the ARV roll-out in 2004 was not a political commitment but rather a political must. Colvin, Fairall, Levin, et al. (2010) state that the South African government's recent policy decision to expand access to HIV care rapidly and "ensure that all health institutions in the country are ready to receive and assist patients and not just a few accredited ARV centres"[5] represents a dramatic and welcome about-turn after years of hesitation and confusion in the country's response to the HIV crisis. In the first 6 years of the antiretroviral therapy (ART) programme, approximately 900,000 people were started on treatment. In the next 2 - 3 years, the government proposes to initiate treatment for another 1.2 million people.[6] The medical and moral imperative for providing this life-saving treatment to all who require it does not need to be defended, but the limited capacity of the public health sector to achieve this scale of increase raises serious questions about the practicality of this objective. This delay in government reaction has not only cost many lives, it has also resulted in a depleted Department of Health at all levels, alienation and distrust amongst the stakeholders, and a vote of no-confidence in the public health care system from the population.

In South Africa, until recently, there was a hostile relationship between the government and the NGO/CSOs and business sectors on the country's response to the pandemic. The reasons for this originate in the political handling of the epidemic during the term of office of President Mbeki. A positive result for the NGO and civil society sector in this dispute was that the international donor world generously started supplying the industry with the financial resources and political support to establish activist, advocacy and human rights platforms (Treatment Action Campaign, AIDS Law Project, etc.) and eventually providing free ARVs in mass roll-out programmes (MSF, PEPFAR, Global Fund), followed by the response of the corporate business sector with prevention and treatment programmes in the workplace (Anglo American, Mercedes Benz, etc.). Some NGOs, like Ndlovu Care Group in 2003, secured private funding to initiate ARV roll-out programmes in the area where they were working, contributing to the discussion of feasible ARV provision in mass programmes with promising long-term results.

Although the Operational Plan for Comprehensive HIV and AIDS Treatment and Care adopted in November 2003 and the HIV and AIDS and STI Strategic Plan for South Africa 2007-2011 signaled a change of direction in the government's AIDS policy, since they centralized conventional biomedical treatment, it was not until the former Deputy-President Ngcuka was appointed as head of the National AIDS Commission in 2006 that relations started to improve between government and civil society. Prior to her nomination, Ngcuka often denounced the government's position. After her nomination, she publicly affirmed that the government believes unequivocally that HIV causes AIDS and that antiretroviral drugs must be the kingpin of the government's response.

In the light of this change in the government's AIDS views and policies, NGOs began to gradually build relationships with the government. One tangible example of this changing policy environment was the increased budget allocation for HIV and AIDS programmes in 2006.

Notwithstanding these signs of change, leaders of civil society continued to be critical of the government. With hindsight, this was because of the wasted opportunities for restraining the pandemic from spreading further, the cumulative effect that this has had on society, and the slow, sometimes obstructive, pace with which acceptable policies were being implemented. NGOs, corporate business, and the government largely continued to operate independently in tackling the HIV/AIDS crisis. Corporate companies started their own HIV prevention, treatment and care programmes in the workplace, including ARV roll-out programmes, because they could no longer tolerate the losses from a human and economic perspective. Civil society organizations applauded the initiative, and the public sector lagged behind. The NGO/CSOs and the business sector at large continued to be sceptical of the government's attitude regarding the pandemic until the fall of the Mbeki government in late September 2008.

Addressing delegates at the 2008 AIDS Vaccine Conference in Cape Town, the new Health Minister, Barbara Hogan, announced a decisive and much-awaited shift in the government's AIDS policy by stating the government's acknowledgement of the generally accepted AIDS science and medicine, and the need to act aggressively in tackling the pandemic.

Both the public and the scientific community recognised in this the end of 10 years of denial that the former leadership of the country exhibited, and a new beginning and an assurance that finally policy is on the right side of science and reality.

After the inauguration of President Zuma, everyone was anxiously awaiting the selection of the new Minister for Health. With the appointment of Aaron Motsoaldi, a medical doctor who has been serving at the provincial level for the last 15 years and as Minister of the Executive Council in Limpopo Province on different portfolios, a man with a low profile but powerful, things are really changing. His office has since taken many decisions that demonstrate a strong dedication, with ambitious targets that force his Department to take action at all levels and implement new legislation, policies and procedures to improve universal access to services. The National Health Department is not ready, however, for a solo attempt at managing the epidemic and servicing the other health care needs in the country.

A major limitation of NGOs is their limited access to resources and therefore their inability to scale up programmes nationally and to sustain programmes over longer periods. The government can utilize its ample public resources and national legitimacy to expand NGO expertise and innovation nationwide. In addition, as partners in the implementation of NSP programmes, NGOs can be the catalysts in the government's pursuit of achieving cost-effective HIV and AIDS interventions. NGOs can employ their implementation and accountability skills to improve efficiencies in public sector service delivery and working conditions. It is the combined effort of government and CSO/NGOs which can drive an increased scaling-up of social development in the rural areas. It is the combined public sector and CSO/NGO response which can deliver the capacity to teach and train, to implement and be accountable for an increased programme implementation.

Lastly, NGOs can use their international networks, with donors and other organisations, to lobby for the government's agenda and to persuade the international community to increase its support for the Global Fund for AIDS, TB and Malaria.

The NGO sector notices at this stage that donor fatigue in response to the South African epidemic is setting in. Donors want to reduce support to NGOs and South Africa in general and would like to change their support to bilateral agreements and technical support rather than direct funding. A coordinated approach amongst donors, NGOs and the government is essential to ensure a smooth transition towards a sustainable long-term solution. The PEPFAR (Presidential Emergency Programme for AIDS Relief) exit strategy transfers all running costs, for the more than half a million patients they initiated on ARVs through NGO support, to the public sector domain by 2013. Although this strategy is politically sound, as the response to the epidemic is a South African governmental responsibility, this strategy further burdens the Department of Health, which is not yet ready for this transition. Resources to take over are not yet in place, and the capacity to manage still has to be created.

The international donor world used major efforts and funding to initiate the donor-supported NGO programmes. These resources can be retained for SA provided that a well orchestrated transition from NGO to public service support is achieved. The phased absorption of the staff and clients from the NGO sector into the public sector will be one of the crucial measures to step up the South African response from emergency to sustainability.

At this stage there is little willingness among the NGO-employed health care and other professionals to migrate into government posts for a variety of reasons, including bureaucracy, structuring of packages, and working conditions. All parties involved will have to determine a strategy to convince staff to migrate to the public sector, otherwise the human resource shortages will once again hamper service delivery.

PEPFAR's initial objective was capacity building in the government sector (hospitals and clinics) and creating access to treatment. The political environment of those days made them divert to the NGO sector, where they built up capacity and provided financial support to this end.

Development cooperation programmes of other donor countries through bilateral agreements or NGO and CSO support are decreasing fast under the smokescreen of the financial recession, changing political climate in donor countries towards development cooperation, and/or the motive that South Africa as a middle-income country should be able to manage its own problems.

The fact of the matter is that a redistribution of wealth has not yet taken place. Some 48% of the population lives below the poverty line of $2 per day (R 462 per month), 48% of the total population is under the age of 15 years, and South Africa has a Gini coefficient of 0.66 (in 2000 it was 0.57). If we take these factors into consideration, the conclusion is that there is a huge inequality that must be addressed while we continue with assistance to life-saving programmes. Stopping assistance for the existing programmes without proper social investment in the public sector will not only mean the loss of lives but also the loss of the investment done over the past few years.

4. The Task and Role of Government

The preamble to the constitution simply states[3]:
   "We, the people of South Africa,
- *recognise the injustices of our past;*
- *honour those who suffered for justice and freedom in our land;*
- *respect those who have worked to build and develop our country; and*
- *believe that South Africa belongs to all who live in it, united in our diversity.*

We therefore, through our freely elected representatives, adopt this Constitution as the supreme law of the Republic so as to:
- *heal the divisions of the past and establish a society based on democratic values, social justice and fundamental human rights;*
- *lay the foundations for a democratic and open society in which government is based on the will of the people and every citizen is equally protected by law;*

- *improve the quality of life of all citizens and free the potential of each person; and*
- *build a united and democratic South Africa able to take its rightful place as a sovereign state in the family of nations."*

This is a phenomenal way of introducing the constitution of South Africa. It shows a commitment towards the people of this country and illustrates the enormous leadership task this country took upon its shoulders. A task which has as its priorities to:
- reconstruct an economy that everybody can be part of;
- establish an education system which is based upon equality and access for all;
- create a quality public health care system that is accessible for all our citizens;
- provide basic public safety for all;
- provide a system to stimulate poverty alleviation;
- protect the beautiful environment.

The main task or role of a responsible government in the fight against the double epidemic of TB and HIV/AIDS is one of committed leadership. Leadership that creates social investment needed to correct the past and to implement comprehensive intervention programmes at all levels, for all citizens.

The mission statement of the National HIV and AIDS and TB programme is to:
a. prevent the spread of HIV, STI and TB infections and
b. to mitigate the impact of the dual HIV and AIDS and TB epidemics on society.

In all of this, the country and the Department of Health are guided by the *HIV and AIDS and STI Strategic Plan for South Africa 2007-2011 and the TB Medium-Term Development Plan.* These plans aim to improve multisectoral participation and to ensure that all spheres of society play an active role in the achievement of the goals of these strategic plans.

The core aims of this programme are to:
- stimulate the government's organization and sense of urgency towards the implementation of the NSP;
- halve the rate of HIV prevalence (new infections not caused by mortality or by migration) by 2011;
- develop a community-based approach with nurses leading the initial treatment;
- seek for new, safer, and cost-effective treatment options;
- make prevention campaigns work better and faster;
- invest in scientific research towards an effective AIDS vaccine;
- lobby the international community to increase support for the Global Fund for AIDS, TB and Malaria;
- promote collective participation of society, government, private sector, civil society and individuals in the fight against HIV/AIDS;
- scale-up mother-to-child prevention programmes and address personal health needs of HIV-positive pregnant women.

At this stage we have identified the following main barriers to achieving the targets set in the NSP 2007-2011 as described above:
- the public health system is over-burdened;

- about a quarter of the total National Health budget is consumed by the HIV and AIDS programmes;
- high mortality rate, especially among women and children;
- increasing resistance towards the drugs we are using due to lack of monitoring and long-term follow-up of our programmes;
- households in the poorest communities are the worst affected (especially in informal settlements).

With these observable challenges in the HIV and AIDS landscape and discourse, it is worthwhile posing the following questions as we are looking for sustainable solutions:

1. What is the nature of the relationship that NGOs and government should have if they are seeking a synergistic partnership?
2. Does government at all layers accept the NGO fraternity as a partner and not as a threat or obstruction?
3. Can the partners, government and NGOs operate independently and interdependently towards an integrated vision?
4. Does government accept that social development and economic development, especially in the rural areas, need to go hand in glove to create a sustainable environment for improved service delivery?

5. The Task and Role of NGOs and CSOs

"Community initiatives must be a priority for our support, because they are the foundation for a sustainable response owned by the people who have the most to lose, the most to gain" (Peter Piot, 2005 [7]). Chapter 9 of the 2006 Report on the global AIDS epidemic[8] states that civil society is made up of ordinary citizens who organize themselves outside of the government and the public service to deal with specific issues and concerns that the normal governmental process cannot address by itself. The report says that societies function more effectively when the state and its citizens engage openly on how policies are formulated and implemented. Civic society therefore includes all the voluntary civic and social organizations and institutions that form the basis of a functioning society as opposed to the force-backed structures of a state and commercial institutions of the market system. The report states that "on the one end of the spectrum they include the women at the village level planting a vegetable garden to feed a family of orphaned children; the nurse who hands out information leaflets on AIDS and TB to fellow churchgoers on Sundays; and the young people in anti-AIDS clubs who distribute condoms to the bars and barber shops in their neighbourhoods. At the other end of the spectrum, civil society includes the development of non-governmental organizations, faith-based organizations, women's groups and other special interest associations, business enterprises and labour unions, private foundations and the media". On page 207 of the report, the following is stated: "Protecting existing human resources across all sectors involved in the AIDS response is a high priority and includes safeguarding the health of people living with HIV. These people are often the backbone of the national response." Further in the report: "Civil society groups play a central role in advocating for greater treatment access, and they also promote greater accountability by monitoring treatment-related activities of governments, donors, and nongovernmental organizations. Enhancing and sustaining the involvement of civil society groups in multisectoral national responses is essential if countries are to get ahead of their epidemics." As well as its work in AIDS-related service provision and advocacy, civil society constitutes a vast reservoir of information and independent expertise for all of the social sectors it works in. In 2005, the amount of money spent on AIDS in low- and middle-income countries was around six times more than what was spent in 2001. The dramatic increase is due in part to the tireless advocacy and activism of civil society organizations at all levels. It still falls short of what is required to get ahead of the epidemic, and a number of civil society organizations continue to work across sectors to focus on mobilizing resources and sustaining the commitment of the international community. Raising the level of funding is as important as ensuring that the money is used effectively to improve people's lives and slow the course of the epidemic.

Civil society organizations or non-governmental organizations bridge the gap between for-profit organisations and governmental service delivery. They perform specialized functions that are either unattractive or not viable enough for the other stakeholders. NGOs are usually formed because of a drive to correct a void or to address a human right. They have the passion to perform and implement, often based on social obligation or frustration because the parties that are supposed to perform those duties lack the will or capacity to do so. NGOs are usually well connected with philanthropical institutions, which enables them to raise funds for the implementation of their strategies. It is one of the primary tasks of NGOs to make government accountable and to convince them of what the delivery inadequacies and shortcomings are. It is also the task of the NGOs to assist the government in its duties when it lacks the capacity to perform.

The main tasks for NGOs are therefore to:
- link philanthropist organisations with the NGOs' visions and missions to fund implementation;
- mobilize community, awareness, engagement, and education;
- advocate for social and other injustices;
- assist government in policy-making;
- assist government in implementing programmes, i.e. direct service delivery;
- act as centres of expertise in their respective fields of operation.

6. The Role of Private Enterprise and Workers' Organizations

Businesses are ideally placed to contribute to the response to the epidemics. They have the capacity to reach millions of workers through workplace AIDS programmes, as well as the communities from which they draw their employees and customers. The 2006 report on Business and AIDS from the World Economic Forum states that an increasing number of companies have AIDS policies in place or plans to introduce them, although the potential remains for a greater contribution to the epidemic response (Bloom, Bloom, & Weston, 2006). Many smaller companies, however, lack the resources to measure the potential impact of HIV on their business, let alone respond. Through corporate social responsibility budgets, businesses are obliged to plough profits back into community development and social responsibility; this has become a major source of cross-fertilisation between NGOs as implementers and the corporate sector as funders.

Employers' organizations have a particular role to play in helping motivate and support smaller, nationally owned, and less well-resourced companies. The Global Business Coalition on HIV/AIDS is a leading and expanding alliance of more than 200 international companies dedicated to responding to the AIDS epidemic. Its aim is to harness the individual and collective power of the world's top corporations to tackle AIDS at the local, national, and international levels. Working to raise awareness and stimulate the business response to AIDS, it created the first international measurement system, the Best Practice AIDS Standard (2007), a quantitative self-assessment tool that measures a company's involvement and guides business strategies for addressing the AIDS pandemic.

Trade unions have also played an important part in the response to HIV. Many unions deal with issues such as pre-employment screening, continuity of employment for people with HIV, provision of sickness benefits and death benefits for dependents. Efforts have also focused on prevention, with the training of union officials and activists as AIDS focal points, peer educators and trainers. In this way, trade unions are helping to extend access to treatment.

7. The Ndlovu Care Group Model as a Model for Stakeholders' Participation

The NCG Rural Advancement Plan (RAP) echoes the Department of Rural Development & Land Reform's vision of vibrant, equitable and sustainable rural communities. The RAP includes the Community Health Awareness Mobilisation & Prevention (CHAMP) Programme, the Autonomous Treatment Centre (ATC), the NCG Child Care Programme, the NCG Monitoring & Evaluation (M&E) Plan, and the NCG Research Consortium. These programme areas cover all aspects addressed in the relevant South African government strategic plans, including the Integrated Sustainable Rural Development Strategy (ISRDP) and the National Strategic Plan 2007-2011.

The RAP covers human and legal rights aspects, not as a separate programme but embedded at a variety of levels, e.g. gender issues, access to grants and official documentation, People Living With Aids (PLWA) support programmes, destigmatisation, and inclusion of PLWA throughout all programmes. The RAP adheres to and respects human and legal rights and is aligned with the Millennium Development Goals, donor strategies and the Three Ones.

The NGO role is to assist the government in its efforts to implement strategic plans and to avoid setting up parallel systems out of frustration or paternalisation. Symbiotic cooperation with the government guarantees the sustainability and value of NGO programmes.

Donors assist temporarily and then leave, and it is therefore imperative that NGOs utilise donor funding as a means and not as an end in itself. The cooperation between the Department of Health and NCG, with the implementation of the Tuberculosis Programme in Moutse since 1997, demonstrates NCG's early efforts to integrate services and to strengthen government delivery. The successful accreditation of NCG in

Limpopo Province and Mpumalanga Province (2009), as one of the first NGOs for HIV-related services in those provinces, further confirms NCG's efforts to make its programmes sustainable through integration into the public sector service delivery systems.

NCG is keen to transfer its RAP across South Africa in partnership with national government departments, civil society partners and private donors, etc. to ensure access to services and achievement for underserved communities and to attain national objectives through the necessary social investment and capacity building.

Through a public-private partnership of the Department of Health & Social Development, at the provincial level, with a locally established CSO and private funders, NCG wants to replicate the model in other rural areas in South Africa. NCG wants to establish the RAP in those rural areas where there is little or no current service delivery. Through this, NCG wants to reinforce district health care and social development strategies and bring care to areas deprived of development where the treatment and service delivery gaps are most prominent. The RAP roll-out strategy involves connecting with local CSOs to establish a reliable relationship with the local representatives of relevant government departments who have a footprint in the community. The private sponsor must have a vested interest to fund the infrastructure needed to implement the RAP, initially an Autonomous Treatment Centre and over time the CHAMP and Child Care Programmes.

NCG has a record of accomplished evidence-based outcomes, and all of these service delivery areas fall within the strategic goals of the South African government. Through the implementation of the RAP, NCG would like to demonstrate how the integration of different government departments can achieve the goals of the Government Action Plan 2008 of alleviating poverty and making a better life for all South African citizens.

To summarize, the holistic RAP for scaling up services and social transformation in underserved communities aims to operate through:

- a partnership between government, private funders, a local NGO and NCG, which together facilitate social development in order to upscale service delivery;
- focused local capacity building, resulting in employment within the local service delivery system and remigration of resources back to rural areas;
- introduction of technology to provide quality services like diagnostics, electronic health records and IT systems;
- system implementation at the programme level to facilitate management, M&E, accountability, information, awareness, communication, and education on relevant issues[9] to promote behavioural change, early detection, early care-seeking behaviour, access to care, and retention in care programmes;
- cost-effective and integrated primary health care (PHC), malaria, TB and HIV/ AIDS care to promote personal well-being and community health in general;
- child care programmes to address the needs and life skills of orphans and vulnerable children (OVC) and women, and to assist in improving the South African public sector service delivery for this group;
- identifying, screening, selecting, developing, and nurturing of individuals to achieve self-actualisation and a long-term orientation towards their future;

- research, monitoring & evaluation to ensure evidence-based interventions and outcomes;
- replicating the NCG model to assist in the strengthening of district health and social welfare service delivery and the upliftment of community systems across South Africa;
- appointment of Ndlovu Care Group as the management entity of the government projects to assist with local capacity-building necessary for improved local governance and programme strengthening for district service systems.

Notes

1. http://www.hsph.harvard.edu/pgda/working.htm
2. Statement from Dr. Peter Piot, UNAIDS Executive Director, on Singing of the "Tom Lantos and Henry J. Hyde Global Leadership Against HIV/AIDS, Tuberculosis and Malaria Reauthorization Act of 2008".
3. TELKOM, Financial Statement 2001-2, cited in Pushing back the frontiers of poverty: Community sector position paper for the Growth and Development Summit (April 2003) (http://www.nedlac.org.za)
4. Pushing back the frontiers of poverty: Community sector position paper for the Growth and Development Summit (April 2003) (http://www.nedlac.org.za)
5. Address by President Jacob Zuma on the occasion of World AIDS Day, Pretoria Showgrounds. 1 December 2009 (http://www.info.gov.za/speeches/2009/09120112151001.htm) (accessed 3 March 2010).
6. Budget Speech 2010 by the Minister of Finance Pravin Gordhan. 17 February 2010. http://www.doh.gov.za/docs/sp/sp0217-f.html (accessed 3 March 2010).
7. Peter Piot: Information Note PCB June 2005; 17th Meeting of the UNAIDS Secretariat Staff Association (USSA), Geneva, 27-29 June 2005.
8. 2006 Report on the Global AIDS Epidemic, Chapter 9: The essential role of civil society. (http://data.unaids.org/pub/GlobalReport/2006)
9. Condomisation, circumcision, child rights, destigmatisation, female empowerment, gender equality, healthy lifestyles, judgemental attitudes

References

Bloom, D.E., Bloom, L.R., & Weston, M. (2006). *Business and Malaria: A Neglected Threat?* World Economic Forum: Global Health Initiative.

Branson, R. (2009). *Business Stripped Bare: Adventures of a Global Entrepreneur.* London: Virgin Books.

Colvin, C., Fairall, F., Levin, S., et al. (2010). Expanding access to ART in South Africa: the role of nurse initiated treatment. *South African Medical Journal, 100* (4), 22-34.

Finlay, J. (March 2007). *Program on the global demography of ageing: The role of health in economic development.* Harvard Initiative for Global Health, Working paper no. 21.

Mbeki, T. (2002). *Africa: Define yourself.* Cape Town: Tafelberg/Mafube.

Chapter 4

Ndlovu Care Group's Approach to Monitoring and Evaluation

Phinah Kodisang[a]

Abstract

Planning, Monitoring, Evaluation and Reporting (PME&R) are key processes in the working cycle of all Ndlovu Care Group (NCG) programmes, helping programme staff to manage, support and improve field practice. Without effective planning, monitoring and evaluation, it would be impossible to judge if work is going in the right direction, whether progress and success can be claimed, and how future efforts might be improved (UNDP, 2009). Similarly, reporting is also a major activity which is undertaken during project monitoring. It is the way in which information about the process and output of activities, and not just the activities, is shared between the stakeholders of the project.[1] This chapter outlines NCG's approach to carrying out the monitoring and evaluation of all programmes, moving from the planning phase to where programmes report on processes and outputs of the project activities. NCG views monitoring and evaluation as a participatory process, which enables capacity building and understanding and applying lessons learned from the programme's and/or projects' experiences. The chapter further outlines steps undertaken by NCG to make M&E operational. Here, M&E is undertaken as part of a process that involves:

1. *assessments* done at the start of the programme (during the planning phase) using participatory evaluations to collect baseline information, in consultation with the community members and stakeholders;
2. *project design*, looking at the problems to be addressed, potential courses of action, and participatory definition and agreement on project concept, consensus about the project objectives and activities with relevant stakeholders;
3. *ongoing monitoring* during implementation;
4. *process and end of programme evaluations* done during the programme and at the end of the programme, respectively; and
5. *reflection* on whether or not NCG programmes are still getting it right, taking into account that situations change, that the needs of project beneficiaries change, and that strategies need to be reconsidered and revised.

---

a. M&E Manager Ndlovu Care Group, Elandsdoorn, South Africa

1. Introduction

Monitoring and evaluation (M&E) provides Ndlovu Care Group (NCG) with better means for learning from past experience, improving service delivery, planning and allocating resources, and demonstrating results as part of accountability to key stakeholders. There is a strong focus within NCG on *results*; hence we have put M&E in place to ensure that we collect appropriate data and achieve evidence-based outcomes. Yet there is often confusion about what M&E entails. The purpose of this chapter is to strengthen awareness and interest in M&E, and to clarify what it entails.

M&E involves systematic data collection of the NCG programme's and project's inputs, outputs, outcomes and impact (Kusek & Rist, 2004).
- *Input:* the resources used for the development intervention, i.e. money, staff, supplies and equipment, etc. invested into each programme and/or project. The people, training, equipment and resources that we put into a project to achieve outputs.
- *Output:* the immediate results achieved by the programme and/or project. For example, outputs may be trained counsellors, clients served and Information, Education and Communication (IEC) materials distributed, which are relevant to NCG programmes and projects. The activities/services we deliver, including HIV/AIDS prevention, care & support services to achieve outcomes.
- *Outcomes:* the intermediate or short-term results achieved by each programme and project. For example, changes in HIV/AIDS-related attitudes, reduction in risk behaviours and adoption of protective behaviours, changes in STI trends are all outcomes measured in NCG programmes and projects such as NAAP (Ndlovu AIDS Awareness Programme).
- *Impact:* the long-term results achieved by the programmes and projects (usually 5-10 years). Good outcomes should lead to major measurable health impacts, reduced STI/HIV transmission and AIDS impact. Long-term effects include impact on HIV/AIDS trends (morbidity and mortality) and sustainability issues.

It is important to understand that inputs lead to outputs, outputs lead to outcomes, and outcomes lead to impacts. Inputs and outputs are short-term indicators, while outcomes and impacts are medium- to long-term measurements.

The M&E core team in NCG includes all support services within NCG in addition to the executive:
1. *M&E*, which is responsible for ensuring, creating and initiating operational plans for comprehensive M&E systems and procedures as well as supporting different departments within NCG to fulfill their M&E responsibilities.
2. *Human Resource Management* (HRM): for NCG's M&E system to function, adequate resources must be available. Thus, the HR department puts in place the necessary conditions, ensuring that there are sufficient human resources and capacities to carry out the activities outlined by the programme design.
3. *Learning and Development* (L&D): since part of the M&E function is to critically reflect on the experiences and the information of the different programmes, L&D ensures that capacity is developed within NCG to improve action.

4. *Finance Department Programme*: M&E reporting is linked with the financial management systems used by NCG. Project financial management is based on flows of information relating to implementation progress, income and expenditure, and other financial functions of the programmes. This is to enable both effective financial management and financial audit functions.
5. *IT-Based Programme and Project Information Management System*: NCG M&E functions are supported by IT-based programme and project information management systems (Health Source). This IT-based programme and project information management system is being further developed for NCG.

2. Monitoring and Evaluation According to NCG

Monitoring

Monitoring is the routine daily assessment of ongoing activities and progress (what is being done). It is an internal function of all NCG programmes carried out by key operations people within the programmes (coordinators, managers and senior managers), and it involves:
– establishing indicators of efficiency, effectiveness and impact;
– setting up systems to collect information relating to these indicators;
– collecting and recording the information;
– analysing the information;
– using the information to inform day-to-day management.

Meticulous monitoring of activities is the foundation for reliable results.

Evaluation

Like monitoring, evaluation also looks at efficiency, effectiveness and impact. In addition, evaluation also aims to determine the relevance and sustainability of a programme. Thus, evaluations carried out by NCG aim to determine the efficiency, effectiveness, impact, relevance and sustainability of all programmes.[2]
   Evaluation involves:
– periodic assessment of overall achievements, what has been achieved, what impact has been made;
– looking at what the programmes intended to achieve, what difference they wanted to make;
– assessing programmes' progress towards what they wanted to achieve, what their impact targets are;
– looking at the strategies of the different programmes, did the programmes have a strategy, were they effective in following their strategies, did each strategy work; if not, why not?
– looking at how it worked, was there an efficient use of resources, how sustainable is the programme's effect, what are the implications for the various stakeholders in the way the programmes work.

A common element of monitoring and evaluation is that they are geared towards learning from what programmes are doing and how well they are doing it, by focusing on (Kusek & Rist, 2004):

- *Efficiency:* A measure of how economically resources or inputs are converted to results. It tells programmes that the input of work is appropriate in terms of the output. This could be input in terms of money, time, staff, equipment, etc.
- *Effectiveness:* A measure of the extent to which programmes achieve the specific objectives they have set. Effectiveness measures how well an indicator or programme competes with other programmes or projects.
- *Impact:* A measure of whether or not the programmes made a difference to the problem situation they were trying to address. In other words, was the strategy employed useful? Impact is usually a long-term indicator that is measured on a large scale. This refers also to positive and negative, primary and secondary, long-term effects produced by a development intervention, directly or indirectly, intended or unintended.

NCG's performance M&E is set up to measure progress towards achievement of the programme[3] and project[4] objectives, prioritising the measurement of all indicators, to achieve the following:

- To monitor the state of programme and project implementation and progress towards objectives. NCG will measure and assess its progress against planned inputs, activities, outputs and outcomes.
- To measure the extent to which NCG is achieving programme and project objectives, such as coverage of care and support of target populations.
- To measure the direct results of the programme and project activities for which managers are accountable and that are used to ensure that the managers are on track with their mandate.

The achievements of the M&E processes form the foundation of reporting. Reporting for donor purposes, reporting for programme evaluation, reporting that leads to critical review of the programme contents, ultimately resulting in improvements and refinement of the programme methods. Reporting also leads to academic review of the programme results with the aim to publish results and make the model known to a wider audience. Donor reporting has as its main aim to inform the donors about programme achievements, efficiency, effectiveness and impact. Combined narrative reports with M&E results and critical observations towards achievements must keep the donors motivated to continue their support so we can continue together to explore new roads in order to develop the environment we work for further.

3. Programme and Project Planning for Monitoring and Evaluation Purposes

Planning refers to the process of setting goals, developing strategies, outlining tasks and schedules to accomplish the goals[5], and most importantly the development of a valid set of indicators. NCG believes in the community development principles of inclusion, empowerment, and community participation. Thus, to design a programme or a project, NCG considers the various contributions that people make in its planning process, no matter what their background or varying abilities. Individual, family, and local needs are acknowledged and addressed, often through informal interaction.

It is very difficult to go back and set up M&E systems once programmes have started running, thus M&E forms part of the planning process. For this purpose, NCG applies six components to its programme and project planning for monitoring and evaluation purposes (see Figure 1).

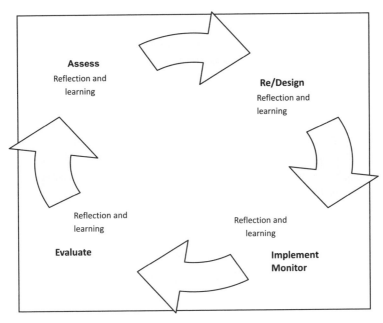

Figure 1: Components of the Programme and Project Management Cycle Planning Process

3.1. Assessment

Assessment refers to the process of defining the 'why' of a proposed programme and/ or project, and it involves scanning the internal and external environments that NCG operates in. NCG assessment processes include identifying community needs and issues through a range of methods, which is instrumental in informing the planning and development of activities and programmes. The external environment is scanned by collecting and analysing information on the community. For this purpose, NCG uses tools such as Participatory Rapid Appraisal (PRA) (Chambers, 1992; Theis & Grady, 1991), CHAMP[6], and PEST[7]. The internal environment is scanned by identifying strengths and weaknesses of the internal NCG resources. The internal scan indicates the in-house capacity and ability of NCG to achieve the new plan. Since the PRA is a qualitative way of doing assessments, it is used as a starting point for understanding the local situation of communities in Moutse East and is a quick, cheap and useful way to gather information. It involves the use of secondary data review, direct observation, semi-structured interviews, key informants, group interviews, games, diagrams, maps and community calendars. In an assessment context, it allows programmes to gather valuable input from those who are supposed to be benefiting from the programme's interventions. It is flexible and interactive. CHAMP, on the other hand, collects information per target area through primary data collection: surveying, either comprehensively or using sampling; or visiting schools and hospitals. The focus lies on NCG's indicators of impact when collecting all this information.

The information collected through these tools is thus used as *baseline data* for programmes and projects (current situation). The baseline data measures what the current status of an environment is before NCG introduces its community intervention programmes and is used as the starting point to measure the achievement of objectives. Baseline data is the information programmes collect about the situation before they do anything. It is the information on which the problem analysis is based. It is very difficult to measure the programme's initiative if we don't know what the situation was when the interventions began. Each programme needs baseline data relevant to the indicators that it has decided will help it measure the impact of its work.

The purpose of conducting assessments is so that NCG can:
– understand the current situation of the communities in context;
– identify opportunities, vulnerabilities (threats), capacities and resources;
– evaluate the feasibility and set priorities for each project and/or programme within the NCG capacity;
– understand the programme scope, logistics, operational resources needed to deliver and budget constraints, to assess the capability of NCG to deliver.

In each programme and project, baseline data documents information relevant to specific interventions of NCG as follows:
1. General demographics such as age, gender, current income, employment status, levels of education, current HIV status and staging of individuals in the community who are enrolled in the clinical programmes (HAART, TB, PMTCT).
2. General information about the situation, e.g. neonatal and under five mortality rates in the area, maternal mortality rates, school enrolment by gender, unemployment rates, and literacy rates. The data collected is required to cover the demographics of each target area. This refers to documented epidemiological information about the target population's (Moutse East) situation at the time the programmes begin working with them.

In summary, *assessment* involves the carrying out of a situation analysis, needs assessment, identification of each programme's overall focus, lessons learned from past programme implementation, taking programme strategies into account and gathering baseline data. It indicates where we are now.

3.2. Programme and Project Re/design

This refers to the process of planning appropriate programme and project strategies using assessment results. Project re/design is an ongoing process over the life of the programme and/or project, which aligns itself according to the following principles:

1. Involvement of all relevant stakeholders in participatory processes of project design.
2. Undertaking a thorough situation analysis.
3. Ensuring and developing a logical project intervention strategy that clearly expresses what will be achieved (goals and purposes) and how it will be achieved (outputs and activities).
4. Identify and agree on cross-cutting objectives (gender, poverty, and empowerment).
5. Planning for long-term capacity development and sustainability to ensure that the project contributes to the empowerment and self-reliance of the local people and organisations.
6. Building in opportunities and activities that support learning and enable adaptation of the project strategy during implementation.

During the initial design phase, NCG conducts the following:
- assessing feasibility, scope and rationale of the project;
- determining the goals and the objectives;
- outlining main project outputs and key activities;
- outlining project implementation process and structures;
- outlining the M&E system;
- developing the budget and specifying staffing levels.

All of the above are documented in a *programme or project description document.*

During the design phase, each programme and project manager, in partnership with relevant stakeholders and the core team, develops a programme and project design document (PDD). The core team is formed of NCG support staff; this includes M&E, L&D, HRM, Marketing and Communication, Finance, IT and executive management. The NCG PDD is a document from which the detailed programme and project plan and the full operational action plan flows. The purpose of the design phase is to ensure that NCG programmes and projects have a logical and strategic plan that prioritises the needs and opportunities identified in the assessment so that the resulting programme or project intervention can be implemented and managed. It involves where we want to go with a plan or what we want to achieve and how we will bridge the gap between baseline and set objectives. NCG ensures that programme and project plans are aligned to the United Nations (UN) Millennium Development Goals (MDGs) as well as to national strategic plans of the government of South Africa.

There are several reasons why the design document is a valuable tool for NCG:
- It communicates NCG's intent to create a new programme or project for relevant stakeholders and the concept behind the new programme or project.

- It explains what needs to be done to progress from baseline to set objectives.
- It outlines the strategy of how this will be achieved.
- It enables NCG executive and relevant funding agencies to give approval to proceed with the intended programme and project intervention.
- It gives operational and stakeholder groups insight into the new programme, allowing them to give timely information and feedback.
- After implementation, the design document is a key part of programme and project curriculum, accountability, and sustainability reviews.

In summary, the *programme and/or project design document* tells us where we are going and what we need to do to achieve the set objectives.

3.3. Implementation & Monitoring

Implementation

Implementation means ensuring that activities leading to the delivery of project or programme outputs are implemented according to NCG principles and standards. Each programme within NCG has a methodology that is applied for carrying out interventions. For clinical services, interventions conform to Batho Pele principles[8], whilst community care services follow the principles of community development as outlined by NCG. The central values on which the development work of each programme within community care services is built are:
- serving disadvantaged and poor people;
- empowering disadvantaged and poor people;
- changing society, not just helping individuals;
- sustainability;
- efficient use of resources.

In terms of the above, our monitoring and evaluation system is designed to give us information about:
- Who is benefiting from what we do? How much are they benefiting?
- Are the beneficiaries passive recipients or does the process enable them to have some control over their lives?
- Are there lessons in what we are doing that have a broader impact than just what is happening in our programmes?
- Can what we are doing be sustained in some way for the long term, or will the impact of our work cease when the programmes stop implementation?
- Are we getting optimum outputs for the least possible amount of inputs?

Monitoring

As indicated before, monitoring is the systematic, ongoing collection and analysis of information as a project and/or programme progresses. It aims to improve the efficiency and effectiveness of a project, programme and/or organisation. It is based on targets set and activities planned during the planning phases of each programme.

Monitoring helps to keep NCG programmes on track, and it lets management know when things are going wrong. If done properly, monitoring becomes an invaluable tool for good management, which provides a useful basis for evaluation. It enables programmes to determine whether the resources available are sufficient and are being well used, whether the capacity within the programmes is sufficient and appropriate, and whether programmes are doing what they planned to do.

Monitoring entails the continuous function that uses the systematic collection of data (qualitative and quantitative) for the purposes of keeping activities on track and measuring progress towards programme objectives.

The use of monitoring provides management and the main stakeholders of NCG with indications of the extent of progress and achievements of objectives as planned and in line with the allocated funds. It provides regular feedback on programme performance. Monitoring helps to identify implementation issues that warrant decisions at different levels of management.

Monitoring tracks the key elements of NCG community care services programmes and projects over time (inputs, outputs, quality of service), as well as community health services. Within community care services, monitoring answers questions such as: To what extent are planned activities being realized? How well are these services provided? Monitoring of e.g. Voluntary Counselling and Testing (VCT) programmes (which cut across community services and community health services) consists of measuring and assessing attendance, return rates and the quality of services (counselling and testing).

In order to answer such questions as 'To what extent are planned activities being realized?', a monitoring system has been put in place which includes day-to-day record-keeping of all activities using tools such as tick sheets (see Appendix 1).

Programmes and projects are monitored by collecting information on a series of input and output indicators. These indicators are collected from a range of instruments or tools, such as the tick sheet. The information is collected daily, as clients undergo a programme, and is aggregated or summed up each month to allow for data analysis.

3.4. Evaluation

Evaluation is the comparison of actual project impacts against the agreed strategic plans. It looks at what programmes have set out to do, at what they have accomplished, and how they accomplished it. Within NCG programmes, evaluation is (i) *formative* (taking place during the life of a project, with the intention of improving the strategy or way of functioning of the project or programme) and (ii) *normative* and (iii) *summative* (drawing conclusions from a completed project – end of project evaluation). Types of evaluations undertaken by NCG and when and why they are conducted are summarized in Table 1.

Table 1: Types of evaluation undertaken by NCG

	Name	When it is conducted	Why it is conducted
Formative	Assessment	Conducted before a programme or project begins and repeated later to understand changes in the programme or project context	**Capacity Development** – building organizational skills, incentives and systems to use evaluation in order to plan and achieve results.
	Feasibility study	Conducted during the design process	
Normative	Baseline	Conducted at the beginning of implementation	**Participation and Empowerment** – evaluations with central objectives to foster participation, learning and empowerment among local stakeholder groups.
	Monitoring	Ongoing during implementation	
Summative	Annual reviews	Conducted annually during implementation	**Programme Improvement** – evaluations focused on improving projects and programmes during the project's life.
	Mid-term evaluations	Conducted in the middle of the project – 3 to 5 years into the project	**Impact Evaluation** – systematic assessment of effects on individuals, households and institutions, caused by any of NCG's development or clinical programmes and/or projects.
	End of programme or project evaluation	At the close of the programme or project	

Evaluation is the systematic assessment of the short-term (outcome) and long-term (impact) results of the programmes and projects. Evaluation answers the questions: To what extent were the objectives of the programme achieved? What short-term and long-term results are observed? What do these results mean? Does the programme make a difference? For example, evaluation of VCT programmes involves assessing risk reduction and changes in sexual behaviours.

NCG evaluations provide information on:
– What worked and what did not work and why?
– What was achieved and what not and why?
– Whether underlying theories and assumptions used in the programme development were valid?
– The relevance, efficiency, effectiveness and sustainability of a programme or project.

In addition, evaluations are used to:
- Guide decision-makers or programme and project managers in reproducing models that succeed;
- Encourage and celebrate the achievements of programmes and projects;
- Assist learning about development.

In summary, during *programme implementation*, monitoring and evaluation ensures continuous tracking of programme progress and adjustment of programme strategies to achieve better goals. At programme completion, in-depth evaluation of programme effectiveness, impact and sustainability ensures that lessons on good strategies and practices are available for designing the next programme cycle.

3.5. Reflection and Learning

Learning is the main reason why NCG programmes and projects monitor their work or conduct an evaluation. By learning what works and what does not, what a programme is doing right and what it is doing wrong, NCG's management is empowered to act in an informed and constructive way. The purpose of learning is to make changes where necessary, and to identify and build on strengths where they exist.

NCG programmes constantly reflect[9] on whether or not they are still getting it right, taking into account that situations change, that the needs of project beneficiaries change, and that strategies need to be reconsidered and revised. Reflections happen in any forum, both formal and informal with key individuals and groups, with project and partner staff and primary stakeholders. In addition, reflections occur in everyday planning, implementation and M&E activities, cutting across all components of the M&E management cycle.

NCG reflection and learning mechanisms entail the following:
- Everyone involved in the programme and/or project implementation monitors at their level;
- Joint planning;
- An enabling environment is created via open leadership and mentoring from the beginning of the programme and/or project;
- Monthly management meetings;
- Participatory evaluations and reviews;
- Periodic and targeted activity reviews;
- Ongoing training to provide new knowledge and skills for the whole team;
- Tailor-made training courses defined by M&E results showing lack of skills or knowledge that needs to be upgraded;
- Ensuring documentation that is systematic and accessible; monthly progress reports that include a section on lessons learnt.

In Figure 2 a summary of the NCG M&E and planning processes is given, which details the steps undertaken for each component.

Assessment (problem analysis)	Develop the design document	Throughout implementation	For evaluation	Reflection requires

- **Collect and review information from primary and secondary sources**
 	
 - Assess together with community members and using the information available from other sources and stakeholders;
 	
 - Find out all information available on the causes of the problems.
 	
 Stakeholder analysis-
 Networking - Linking, forming alliances, collaborating and working with individuals, groups, other agencies, government and business are crucial, with interaction between formal and informal methods to achieve connections within the local communities.
 	
 Write assessment report
	The results of PRA* are developed to intervention ideas
	
	 - Drawing a plan to address related health and social issues identified in the target area in cooperation with responsible government (local) and other organisations, and planning and implementing measures and activities which the community participate in.
	
	 - These activities will be measured and reported to the community and to other stakeholder organisations.
	
	 - Further activities will be undertaken as needed, and as knowledge and capacities to plan measures and implement the plans increase.
	
	 - **For monitoring; construct the logical framework:**
	  - Develop objectives, outcomes and indicators
	  - Baseline programme and project indicators
	  - **Write M&E plan**
	  - Data collection plan
	  - Data collection tools and responsibilities
	  - Frequency of data collection
		- Build relationships; then introduce new ideas, showing how they meet identified needs.
		
		 - Involve as many community people as possible in all activities from the start.
		
		 - Train people in locally acceptable ways (e.g. methods, facilities). Train trainers who can train others. Involve local leadership.
		
		 - Cooperate with government departments and other relevant stakeholders
		
		 Monitoring
		
		 - Progress monitoring: The project manager must collect data monthly to monitor project progress against the plan to ensure progress remains within acceptable limits
		
		 - Performance monitoring: Improvement in performance can only be realistically achieved when management is properly informed about current performance - monthly report to management about progress made and challenges faced.
		
		 Write M&E report monthly
			- Develop ToR** for the evaluation.
			
			 - Ensure data collection methods and tools are developed
			
			 - Ensure that evaluation of projects is generally done towards the end of the project implementation and should be included along with monitoring in project design.
			
			 - Ensure projects are evaluated in terms of impact.
			
			 - Project evaluations should include a participatory component.
			
			 - Ensure evaluation report is compiled and present evaluation findings to partners, using appropriate methods
				NCG and the relevant stakeholders to reflect together on, and evaluate the project, its outcomes and conclusions and prepare a report on this. The reflection may be done in a workshop mode.
				
				 - Lessons learnt should be used to improve future programming or redesign the current programme
				
				 - Lessons learnt are important to assist others benefit from NCG's experiences and successes

Figure 2: NGG´s M&E and planning processes (* PRA: Participatory Rapid Appraisal, ** ToR: Terms of Reference)

3.6. *Reporting*

Reporting is done using a narrative report (see Appendix 1) and a data and financial report. The data reports are based on the log frames of the different programme tick sheets.

4. Conclusion

The design of useful, participatory and results-oriented M&E is more than just matching stakeholder information needs with particular methods, approaches and models, although this is important in itself. M&E processes should be conceived of as involving continuous and inclusive assessment, reflection, dialogue, learning, feedback and action on multiple levels. This therefore requires that NCG creates an enabling environment where stakeholders, including donors, see each other as partners with the common ultimate purpose of achieving development and successful clinical results. It is for this reason that NCG recognises the importance of M&E and acknowledges that M&E's use does not start (or stop) once reports are generated. While NCG M&E processes address issues identified locally as meaningful, our hope is that the results will prompt stakeholders to act on what they come to know as a result of the feedback received from assessments and ongoing monitoring of programmes and projects. Unless M&E processes ensure stakeholders are empowered (and resourced) to act on their knowledge, the process is thwarted.

Notes

1. http://www.scn.org/cmp/hemon.htm
2. http://www.unfpa.org/monitoring/toolkit/defining.pdf
3. A time-bound intervention, consisting of one or more projects that co-ordinate to achieve a desired programme goal. A *programme* cuts across sectors or themes, uses a multi-disciplinary approach, involves multiple partners [and institutions], and may be supported by several different funding sources (World Vision Development Resources Team, 2005).
4. A *project* is a series of activities (investments) that aim at solving particular problems within a given time frame and in a particular location. The investments include time, money, human and material resources. Before achieving the objectives, a project goes through several stages. Monitoring should take place at and be integrated into all stages of the project cycle (http://www.scn.org/cmp/hemon.htm). It may involve multiple partners [and institutions] and may be supported by several different funding sources, but often is supported by a single donor.
5. http://www.investorwords.com/3710/planning.html
6. Community: Care Health Awareness Mobilisation Prevention: (CHAMP) represents all the community care programmes in the NCG portfolio.
7. Political, Environmental, Socio-Economic, Technological trend scan to determine the uncontrollable influences on a project.
8. http://www.socdev.ecprov.gov.za/Documents/Principles_of_Batho_Pele.pdf
9. Reflection is a periodic process of taking time to look back and analyse the data collected, then look forward to consider its implications for programmes and projects. Reflection is a process that brings people together to learn about their work and themselves, and in doing so develop as individuals and as an organisation. Reflection is a proactive process that reviews what has happened and plans future learning before an experience takes place.

References

Chambers, R. (1992). *Rural Appraisal: Rapid, Relaxed, and Participatory.* Institute of Development Studies Discussion Paper 311. Sussex: HELP.

Kusek, J.Z., & Rist, R.C. (2004). *Ten Steps to a Results-Based Monitoring and Evaluation System: A Handbook for Development Practitioners, 289,* p. 223-229. Washington, D.C. World Bank.

Theis, J. & Grady, H. (1991). *Participatory Rapid Appraisal for Community Development.* London: Save the Children Fund.

UNDP (2009). *Handbook on Planning, Monitoring and Evaluating for Development Results.* New York: United Nations Development Programme, Office of Evaluation and Strategic Planning.

Appendix 1

Monthly Narrative Management Report

Submitted by:
Submission date:

1. Achievements and Milestones

   Report achievements against the set targets within programme activities of the applicable reporting month.

   Report on milestones which include impact achievements facilitated by either the programme or staff contribution. Think outside the box.

   1.1   ACHIEVEMENTS

   1.2   MILESTONES

2. Challenges and Limitations

   Report on programme and financial management challenges that restricted the programme from achieving its targets. Management has full control over these challenges.

   Report on programmatic limitations independent of management's control.

   2.1   CHALLENGES

   2.2   LIMITATIONS

3. SWOT Analyses

   Below you will find a SWOT analysis. The Strengths and Weaknesses have to do with the programme itself, the Opportunities and Threats are independent of the programme.

   3.1   STRENGTHS

   3.2   WEAKNESSES

   3.3   OPPORTUNITIES

   3.4   THREATS

4. Action Plans and Target for different activities

   If action is required ensure linkage between your action plan(s) and what has been reported above. Each action plan includes a preparation, implementation, and evaluation stage.

   If more action plans are required, copy paste template for action plan 1.

ACTION PLAN 1

Step	Description	Target	Period
	PREPARATION STAGE		
1			
2			
3			
4			
5			
	IMPLEMENTATION STAGE		
6			
7			
8			
9			
10			
	EVALUATION STAGE		
11			
12			
13			
14			
15			

CHAMP DAILY TICK SHEET

Name of Counsellor _____   Event _____   Date: ..../........../20......

Record no.	Client's Age	Client's Sex		Services offered			HIV test done		Test Result		CD4 Count	Post test counselling		Client intends to share results with partner		Condoms given					# T-shirts = VCT given	# IEC mat. Given	Referral		
		M	F	Info only	Couns. Only	Full VCT	Yes	No	Pos	Neg		Yes	No	Yes	No	Yes = Demo	Yes ≠ Demo	No	CDs # Avail	# CDs given			Yes	No	Where to?
1																									
2																									
3																									
4																									
5																									
6																									
7																									
8																									
9																									
10																									
11																									
12																									
Totals																									

Programme supervisor _____ Date _____

Chapter 5

Development of Evidence-Based Research

Anke Gosling[a], *Adri Vermeer*[b]

Abstract

This chapter provides a description of applied research methodology and the importance of a 'Centre of Expertise' for the future replication of the Ndlovu Care Group (NCG) model. NCG identifies and designs research topics for the evaluation of all aspects of the NCG model and provides evidence-based results to prove the potential effectiveness, impact, efficiency and possibility to replicate the model in rural settings. Research data are needed to ensure valid and reliable outcomes of the tested interventions.

1. Introduction

This chapter describes the applied research methodology employed at Ndlovu Care Group (NCG) under the supervision of the newly established Ndlovu Research Consortium (NRC). NCG developed a replicable model for scaling up services in communities in limited-resource settings. The NCG model consists of a number of health and community development programmes and is implemented in underserved rural areas of South Africa. These NCG programmes operate on three different levels: community-based, household and individual levels that represent all age groups in a community. Research activities on all these levels ensure that NCG can prove that it achieves its set of objectives and measure the extent to which the objectives are achieved. Research outcomes are used to improve the monitoring and evaluation of the programmes, and to localise and align indicators with the Millennium Goals and the SA National Strategic Plans of the diverse government departments. Research outcomes are also used to share experiences, contribute to the academic field and prove the effectiveness of the NCG model.

Over the last ten years, NCG conducted several research projects in co-operation with foreign and national universities, in particular in the disciplines of social and behavioural sciences, health sciences and medical sciences. This book provides a programme research summary at the end of several chapters, with background information, research objectives, data collection and analysis, main results and the authors' suggestions for future NCG research.

---

a. Research Manager, Ndlovu Care Group, Groblersdal, South Africa
b. Professor emeritus of Special Education, Faculty of Social and Behavioural Sciences, Utrecht University, The Netherlands

Research to establish evidence-based practices is fundamental for the replication of the NCG model in rural South Africa. 'In evidence-based practice the evidence in question is of a particular nature or type, viz. that acquired from well-controlled experimental trials which indicate the effects and effect sizes of an intervention' (Cohen, Manion & Morrison, 2000; p. 394). The development and implementation of international standard research plans require diverse and specialised knowledge to accurately measure the effectiveness, efficacy and impact of the complete NCG model. This has led to the establishment of the Ndlovu Research Consortium within NCG. Research facilitation became an important part of the operational managers' duties, and all managers attended a course in Applied Research Methodology that was developed specifically for NCG management by Utrecht University, the Netherlands. NCG utilises applied research methodologies primarily for the professional consolidation, understanding, development and advancement of programme managers.

2. Applied Research Methodology

'The research techniques, procedures and methods that form the body of research methodology are applied to the collection of information about various aspects of a situation, issue, problem or phenomenon so that information gathered can be used in other ways – such as for policy formulation, administration and the enhancement of understanding of a phenomenon' (Kumar, 2005; p. 9). The results are used to understand a phenomenon/issue or to adapt a programme or situation.

For NCG programmes, the focus of an evaluation could be either process- or product-oriented. With regard to the focus of this chapter, namely research relevant for programme evaluation, process-oriented research investigates whether the execution of a programme is being done according to the intended plan, whether there is consistency between the aspects of the programme, and whether the programme resulted in the expected outcomes. Product-oriented research focuses on the establishment of the theoretically tested relationship between an intervention and its outcomes. This explains the difference between *monitoring & evaluation* (M&E) as a process-oriented approach and *empirical research* as a product-oriented approach of programme evaluation. 'Without effective planning, monitoring and evaluation, it would be impossible to judge if work is going in the right direction, whether progress and success can be claimed, and how future efforts might be improved' (see Chapter 4). 'Within empirical research, you work within a framework of a set of philosophies or theories, use methods that have been tested for validity and reliability, and attempt to be unbiased and objective. Research must as far as possible, be controlled, rigorous, systematic, valid and verifiable, empirical, and critical' (Kumar, 2005; pp. 6-7).

2.1. Research Designs and Methods

This section discusses the most relevant types of applied research to be used at NCG. Applied research involves using knowledge, philosophies, theories, instruments and methods developed in other types of research, e.g. fundamental research, philosophical studies, exploration and testing of a theory, construction of classification systems or measuring instruments. The application of the theoretical and/or instrumental knowledge concerns a practical context, e.g. health care, clinical settings, education, community development. Several types of applied research could be relevant for research activities to be carried out within the NCG context.

Literature Studies

A *literature study* is always the first step in any research project. Literature studies can be classified as either a literature review or a meta-analysis. *Literature reviews* are comprehensive and include all valid papers relevant for the topic being studied. Details concerning the methods used and main results of the studies are critically presented (Bowling, 2002). An example of such a study can be found in the study into *'Influences on the Nutritional Status of Children'* carried out in the Elandsdoorn township area in Limpopo Province, where NCG has established a number of nutritional units (de With, Wouters & Jongmans, 2008). *Meta-analysis* is based on high-level statistics. This technique uses statistical methods to combine results from different studies and analyses these results to obtain a single observation of the aggregated data (Bowling, 2002). Up to now, no meta-analyses have been performed by NCG.

Descriptive Research

Next, several *descriptive studies* are carried out. Descriptive research in general systematically describes a situation, problem, phenomenon, programme or services, or provides information about communities, or describes attitudes towards an issue (Kumar, 2005). In the book *Health care in Rural South Africa: An Innovative Approach* (Vermeer & Tempelman, 2008), examples of this type of research can be found (pp. 115-124; 175-200; 201-224).

Another type of descriptive research is epidemiological research. *'Epidemiology* is a study of the distribution, determinants and frequency of diseases in human populations'* (Bowling, 2002; p. 63). For its care policy, NCG refers to several South African epidemiological studies, in particular with respect to HIV/AIDS. Within the organisational framework of NCG, an epidemiologist is appointed to carry out this kind of research in a rural area where a new satellite of NCG will be developed.

Qualitative Empirical Research

Also the distinction between *qualitative* and *quantitative research* is relevant for NCG. Qualitative research describes the variation in phenomena, situations or attitudes, whereas quantitative research quantifies the variation (Kumar, 2005*).*

Qualitative empirical research can be conducted by means of case studies, interviews, observations, and content analysis.

A *case study* is a research method that focuses on a single or small number of cases, e.g. a patient or a hospital. It is a valuable method for complex cases or settings and is useful in the exploratory, early stages of research (Bowling, 2002). An example of such a study is the one by Marcus (2008), *To Live a Decent Life: Bridging the Gaps* (between AIDS-related illness and death in children, their families and communities), carried out on behalf of the AIDS Office of the Southern African Catholic Bishop's Conference (SACBC) in Pretoria.

Unstructured interviews aim to look into in-depth responses to obtain true meanings and untangle the complexity of attitudes, behaviours and experiences (Bowling, 2002). An example of such a qualitative descriptive study is the one by De Waal (2008), *'Turning the Tide: A Qualitative Study of ARV Treatment Programmes'*, also carried out on behalf of the AIDS Office of the Southern African Catholic Bishop's Conference (SACBC) in Pretoria.

Qualitative observation of behaviours, actions, activities and interactions is a tool to understand people's answers to questions in more depth and can help to elucidate complex situations. This is a research method in which the researcher systematically watches, listens and records the phenomenon of interest, e.g. verbally or by means of pictures or drawings (Bowling, 2002).

Content analysis presents qualitative data in a categorised manner. Data are collected by means of an interview, a questionnaire or an observation method and coded by category. The coded data are analysed and presented (Bowling, 2002). Klop, Gardeniers, Tempelman, et al. (2008) used such a method to explore a 'Conceptual Framework for Weight-for-Age', a model to identify risk factors for underweight children in a rural area in South Africa.

Quantitative Empirical Research

Quantitative empirical research can be descriptive/explorative, involving construction of a measuring instrument and hypothesis testing. Descriptive/explorative research can be conducted as a survey, interview, questionnaire, observation or test.

Descriptive surveys are carried out to describe populations, examine associations between variables and establish trends. A cross-sectional approach is done at one point in time and gives a description of data. Longitudinal surveys are conducted at more than one point in time to analyse cause and effect relationships. If you repeat a survey at another time or place, the results can be compared (Bowling, 2002). Examples of such surveys are the studies of Barth, Tempelman and Hoepelman (2009), a long-term virological follow-up of HIV-infected patients, and those of Barth, Tempelman, Smelt, et al. (2009), a long-term follow-up into the effects of Anti-Retroviral Treatment of children with HIV/AIDS.

Structured or semi-structured interviews and *questionnaires* allow researchers to count answers, leading to quantitative data for analysis. Examples are the KAPP surveys carried out within the Community Health Awareness Mobilisation & Prevention (CHAMP) programme to establish risk behaviour and perceptions regarding stigmatisation towards HIV/AIDS.

Quantitative observations can be structured by means of a checklist, categories to check, or rating scales, leading to quantitative data (Bowling, 2002). An example of using an observation instrument to describe the interaction between a childcare worker and a disabled child can be found in the book by Vermeer & Tempelman (2008), in the part where research in Sizanani Children's Home, a residential facility for children with physical disabilities in Bronkhorstspruit, is described (pp. 295-312; 313-330).

The *construction of a measuring instrument* is the operationalization of a theoretical concept. It is very important to understand the concept behind indicators and measurements. The concept needs to be translated into measurable terms, from chosen indicators to measurable variables (Kumar, 2005). In NCG research into the effects of the Ndlovu AIDS Awareness Programme (NAAP), a lot of attention is paid to the construction of a reliable and valid questionnaire to measure the effects of the programme on behaviour change (in particular condom use) and to measure the factors (determinants) influencing the expected behaviour. The scales of this questionnaire were based on the Planned Behaviour Model of Ajzen (1991) (see Vermeer & Tempelman, 2008; pp. 159-174; 175-200).

Hypotheses are important for clarification, specification and focus on a research question. It is crucial with hypothesis testing that all aspects of the study – design, sampling procedure, method of data collection, data analysis, statistical procedures or conclusions – are correct. This results in proper verification of the hypothesis (Kumar, 2005). Using hypothesis testing as a research design requires the use of a theory which has proven validity for the research to be carried out. The research hypotheses have to be formulated in such a way that the relationships between the variables to be investigated could be predicted on the basis of the underlying theory. With respect to NCG research, there are not that many theories yet which have proven validity for NCG research. This implies that NCG research mostly has an exploratory nature: based on a theory proved to be applicable elsewhere, at best it can be expected that a relationship exists (or not).

Intervention Research

For NCG, a highly relevant type of research is intervention research. It aims at the establishment of the outcomes of a programme. There are so many types of experimental designs for intervention research that we will only discuss three which are used in intervention research: a pre-, true- and quasi-experimental design.

The *pre-experiment* uses a method to test cause and effect relationships between independent and dependent variables of mostly only an experimental group and sometimes also an equivalent control group investigated systematically under conditions that are identical in order to minimize variation between them (Bowling, 2002). 'The *true experiment* also requires the randomisation of participants to experimental and control groups' (Bowling, 2002; p. 216). In the NCG situation this is almost impossible. Thus, the most commonly used design is a *quasi-experimental design*. It has the properties of both pre- and true-experimental studies (Kumar, 2005). There are a lot of types of quasi-experimental designs (Cook & Campbell, 1979). Roughly, they can be divided into ones with and without a control group. The application of designs with a control group is not that feasible. It is ethically unacceptable to deprive a person in need of treatment, education or training for research aims. This implies that a quasi-experimental design without a control group is mostly used. The best solution then is for a person under intervention to act as his/her own control. Then, the best fitting design is a 'baseline-intervention follow-up' design. An example of such a design is used in the study into the effects of a training programme on children with physical disabilities living in a residential setting, Sizanani Children's Home, in Bronkhorstspruit (Vermeer, Wijnroks & Magyarszeky, 2008).

2.2. Research Instrument

Validity and reliability are important issues in all research processes. 'The validity ensures correct procedures are applied to find answers to a research question. The reliability refers to the quality of the measurement procedure that provides repeatability and accuracy' (Kumar, 2005; p. 6). NCG research often requires the development of new or adapted research instruments due to the socio-cultural differences between the setting where most measuring instruments are developed and the NCG settings where a specific measuring instrument will be used. There are several types of validity and reliability. The most relevant for NCG research are mentioned in Appendix 1.

Validity

An important type of validity is 'content validity'. Content validity concerns the assessment of the items of an instrument. This means that 'each aspect should have similar and adequate representation in the questions and items' (Kumar, 2005; p. 155). An attempt was made to guarantee the content validity of the questionnaire constructed in the above-mentioned study into the effects of NAAP by taking existing questionnaires based on the Ajzen model with proven reliability and validity as a starting point (see Vermeer & Tempelman, 2008; pp. 159-174; 175-200).

For the definition of other types of validity, the literature about research methodology has to be consulted (Kumar, 2005; Bowling, 2002; Baarda & de Goede, 2008).

Reliability

Questionnaires are very often used in NCG research. The reliability of a questionnaire can be estimated by means of Cronbach's alpha. This procedure is based on all possible correlations between all the items within the scale of the instrument (Bowling, 2002). For example, the research to establish the determinants of the participation in Voluntary Counselling and Testing (VCT) (Tempelman & Vermeer, 2009) was measured by means of a questionnaire based on the Planned Behaviour Model of Ajzen (1991). Cronbach's alpha for the five scales of this questionnaire proved to be acceptable to good (.59-.88).

For the definition of other types of reliability, the literature about research methodology has to be consulted (Kumar, 2005; Bowling, 2002; Baarda & de Goede, 2008).

2.3. Data Analysis

Many statistical procedures are used to analyse the collected data. Depending on the level of measurement of a measuring instrument, viz. nominal, ordinal, interval or ratio, different statistical analyses are possible. The choice of a statistical technique is based on the calculations of frequencies, differences, and cohesion/correlations/relationships. There are several computer programmes such as SPSS, SAS (quantitative data) and WINMAX (qualitative data) for these statistical procedures. Data are extracted from the database and imported into one of these statistical programmes.

2.4. A Master Class for the NCG Management

The need for evidence-based results to prove the replicability of the NCG model requires extra skills and a new way of thinking for operational managers. It is very important that all aspects of a research are properly thought through and incorporated in a programme research plan before embarking on a project. This ensures the validity of the methodology for obtaining answers to the research question(s) in an unbiased and objective manner. In order to achieve this, a research proposal has to be formulated. It must include *what* you are proposing to do, *how* you plan to proceed and *why* you selected the proposed research design. NCG management needed this shift in thinking and a new set of tools to apply research as part of their duties. An in-service training 'Master Class' programme was developed and presented over a period of two years (Vermeer, 2008). During this training, methodology and practical assignments are discussed and presented. The main goal of this master class was the development of proposals for research to evaluate the products and processes of NCG programmes. After one year of teaching, one year of intervision followed. During these intervision classes, research proposals and initial actions to take were discussed.

All phases of research are discussed in detail during the master class programme (listed below to give an overview of specific aims for managers attending the master class):
– to indicate the purpose of the research;
– to formulate sound research questions;
– to specify the practical and scientific relevance;
– to describe a frame of reference (theoretical);
– to develop a design for the programme/project research;
– to indicate the means of data collection;
– to store and process the data;
– to analyse the data;
– to describe the results of a specific project research (report, article);
– to draw conclusions from the results;
– to evaluate the results of the research (discussion);
– to formulate recommendations for practical applications and further research;
– to cite references (literature) correctly.

3. Development of a Research Agenda

NRC drafted a research agenda for the next five years to include the different research proposals. A research proposal informs all parties of the conceptualisation of the total research process, and examines its suitability and validity (Kumar, 2005). The guidelines of a research proposal set by NCG (see Appendix 1) provide a framework for writing a research proposal. It should be written in an academic style. It must contain appropriate references in the body of the text and a bibliography at the end. Certain requirements in the guidelines for a research proposal are not applicable to all types of proposed research; therefore, the researcher has to be selective regarding what is needed for a specific research proposal. The guidelines are based on those described in the book, *Second edition of Research Methodology – A Step By Step Guide for beginners*, by Ranjit Kumar (2005). At NCG, a programme research plan and the proposals for a specific research project regarding an NCG programme are evaluated by the Ndlovu Research Consortium (NRC) before approval. It will be judged according to this frame of reference and its interest and/or applicability to NCG.

New research plans and projects within NRC are often developed in co-operation with the Epidemiology and M&E departments, depending on the type of research to be carried out. The role of the NRC is to assess the submitted research plans and proposals on content, research methodology and comprehensiveness according to the guidelines. The NRC will evaluate the content and applicability of the research to ensure its long-term goals (outcomes & impacts) within the NCG programmes are met (see Chapter 4).

When a research plan or proposal has been approved by the NRC and all other stakeholders, it will be submitted to an ethics committee connected to a local university or SAMA (South African Medical Association) for final approval before the research is started. Ideally, the NRC will develop its own ethics committee in time.

4. Relationships with Universities

In 2002, a relationship was established between NCG and the Faculty of Social and Behavioural Sciences of Utrecht University in the Netherlands. This fruitful relationship has resulted in several research projects (Vermeer & Tempelman, 2008). This cooperation was formalised by the establishment of the Ndlovu Research Consortium which aims at scientific cooperation between several parties, viz. NCG, Utrecht University, UNISA (University of South Africa) and the University of Pretoria (see Chapter 1).

In this context, MSc students from Dutch universities have developed research proposals according to the NCG and university guidelines and applied for a student position at NCG. Literature studies, tool development and other preparations are done at the university under the guidance of their individual supervisors while the data collection takes place in the rural areas of South Africa. So far, mainly quantitative research has been conducted, but more and more qualitative research is necessary to look at concepts and problems in depth. Questionnaires are developed and tested before the actual research is conducted. Interviews, observations, focus groups and patient records provide data to answer many research questions. Theories are studied and used as a frame of reference to examine associations and relationships between influencing factors and to look at behavioural change in particular. After data collection, a preliminary analysis is done and presented to programme management and programme staff. Within two months after data collection, a final scientific article must be written about the results. Management has to be able to translate these results into operational changes and improvements, or develop a new research plan for further investigation concerning the matter. The MSc students then finalize this research project and use it for their graduation project.

The theoretical framework used most often for social behaviour change (e.g. participation in a programme, showing health-oriented behaviour) is the Theory of Planned Behaviour (TPB). TPB focuses on the theoretical constructs that predict individual motivational factors as determinants of the likelihood of performing a specific behaviour (Montano & Kasprzyk, 1990). According to the theory, a person's behaviour is a result of his/her intention to perform the particular action (Azjen, 1991), and this intention is influenced by three factors: the attitude towards the behaviour, the perceived attitudes of important others (subjective norm) and the perceived behavioural control (Fisher & Fisher, 200).

In the medical field a PhD research project evaluated the clinical results of NCG's public health interventions, resulting in several publications (Barth, 2010). Those results showed the importance of documenting and evaluating the work done. The results became tools for the NCG executives to advocate for improvements in the national guidelines to the benefit of the community in South Africa at large.

Utrecht University developed this North-South Policy within its Africa Research Cooperation: as a university from the Northern hemisphere, they want to connect to a university in the Southern hemisphere in order to, synergistically, strengthen programmes in the field in Africa. Utrecht University, the University of Pretoria, UNISA and Ndlovu Care Group are implementing this policy in South Africa. NRC will coordinate policy implementation through twinning of students from UP, UNISA and UU.

5. Centre of Expertise

NCG is developing an applicable and replicable model for scaling up services in underserved communities, and this strategy demands evidence-based interventions to be successful. Evidence-based interventions to measure the success of the complete NCG model require expertise in a variety of disciplines, e.g. research methodology, health science, social and behavioural science, psychology, epidemiology, internal medicine, infectious diseases, virology, education, economics and statistics. To conduct these complex research activities demands a certain level of research skills, researchers and funds. NCG as a 'Centre of Expertise' has to provide the evidence supporting the NCG model for advancing rural communities. NRC will, through research, attempt to prove the effectiveness and need for future replication of the NCG model in underserved populations.

6. Implications for NCG

Several implications for NCG could be derived from the research message of this chapter:
1. Research priorities have to be formulated within the fields of expertise of the NCG staff. The following recommendations could function as a guideline for such a priority list.

2. Extensive descriptions have to be made of the contents of the NCG programmes. A first draft of the existing NCG programmes is provided in Parts Two and Three of this book. An example of a well-elaborated programme description is provided in the 'Manual Training for AIDS Awareness' (Rood, van der Schaaf, Wubbels, et al., 2008).

3. Epidemiological surveys have to be carried out before a new NCG satellite can be implemented, including assessment of the population's needs.

4. The mission of NCG concerns improving the quality of life of people living in the rural areas where NCG is active. This implies all kinds of changes on the individual, family and community levels by means of well-designed interventions. To establish the proof of the success of these interventions, intervention research has to be carried out. Therefore, it could be stated that intervention research has to be one of the main types of research carried out by NCG staff members.

5. An immediate consequence of the execution of intervention studies is that they must be followed by longitudinal surveys to establish the long-term impact of the NCG interventions.

6. To develop a common drive within the organisation for the use of M&E and research strategies, regular meetings of the NCG staff have to be held to learn about the proposed M&E and research methods and to discuss the implications of research which has been carried out. Such meetings could be considered a kind of in-service training.

7. It is evident that not all staff members have to become researchers. Staff members need to act as the facilitators of research activities. At very least, they must be able to set up IT-based client registration and follow-up systems which could be used as a database for more advanced research. Academically trained staff members have to be able to make research plans in cooperation with the NCG Research Consortium.

8. Every year a report of NCG research activities and outcomes has to be published.

References

Azjen, I. (1991): The Theory of Planned Behaviour. *Organizational Behaviour and Human Decision Processes, 50,* 179-211.

Baarda, D.B. & de Goede, M.P.M. (2008). *Basisboek Methoden en Technieken. Handleiding voor het opzetten en uitvoeren van onderzoek.* Groningen: Stenfert Kroese.

Barth, R.E. (2010), *Treating HIV in Rural South Africa: Successes and Challenges.* Dissertation. Utrecht: University Medical Centre Utrecht.

Barth, R.E., Tempelman, H. & Hoepelman, I.M. (2009) Long-term virological follow up of HIV-infected adults in rural South Africa. *International Aids Society (IAS).* Cape Town: 19-22 July 2009, *abstract no: CDB084.*

Barth, R.E., Tempelman, H., Smelt,E. Hoepelman, I.M., Wensing, A.M. & Geelen, S. (2009). Long Term Follow Up of ART in a Pediatric Cohort in Rural South Africa; Virologic Failure on First Line Treatment. *Interscience conference of antimicrobial agents and chemotherapy (ICAAC),* 11-15 Sept 2009, *poster no: H-911*

Bowling, A. (2002). *Research methods in health: Investigating health and health services.* Second edition. Maidenhead: Open University Press, McGraw Hill Education.

Cohen, L., Manion, L. & Morrison, K. (2000). *Research Methods in Education*. London: Routledge Falmer.

Cook, T.D. & Campbell, D.T. (1979). *Quasi-Experimentation. Design & Analysis Issues for Field Settings*. Boston: Houghton Miffin Company.

Fisher, J.D., & Fisher, W.A. (2000). Theoretical approaches to individual-level change in HIV risk behaviour. In: J.L. Peterson & R.J. Diclemente (Eds.), *Handbook of HIV Prevention, AIDS prevention and Mental Health* (pp. 3-55). New York, NY: Kluwer Academic/Plenum Publishers.

Klop, E., Gardeniers, A., Tempelman, H. et al. (2008). A Conceptual Model for Weight-for-Age among Children Aged 1-8 Years. In: Vermeer, A. & Tempelman, H.A. (Eds.), *Health Care in Rural South Africa: An Innovative Approach* (pp. 91-100). Third edition. Amsterdam: VU University Press.

Kumar, R. (2005). *Research Methodology – A step-by-step guide for beginners. Second edition*. SAGE Publications.

Marcus, T. (2008). To Live a Decent Life: Bridging the Gaps. In: Vermeer, A. & Tempelman, H.A. (Eds.), *Health Care in Rural South Africa: An Innovative Approach* (pp. 433-468). Third edition. Amsterdam: VU University Press.

Rood, S., van der Schaaf, M., Wubbels, T., Kanselaar, G., Vermeer, A., van der Lubbe, K., Tempelman, H. & Slabbert, M. (2008). *Training for AIDS Awareness, Manual*. Pretoria: Health & Medical Publishing Group (HMPG).

Montano, D.E. & Kasprzyk, D. (1990). The theory of reasoned action and the theory of planned behaviour. *Health Behaviour and Health Education, 4,* 67-95.

Tempelman, H. & Vermeer, A. (2009). An AIDS Awareness Programme in Rural South Africa to Promote Voluntary Counselling and Testing. In: Lagerwerf, L., Boer, H. & Wasserman, H. (Eds.), *Health Communication in Southern Africa: Engaging with Social and Cultural Diversity* (pp. 241-260). Amsterdam: Rozenberg Publishers/Pretoria: UNISA Press.

Vermeer, A. (2008). *Manual Applied Research Methodology for Disability Care*. Utrecht: Vereniging Gehandicaptenzorg Nederland.

Vermeer, A., & Tempelman, H.A. (Eds.) (2008). *Health Care in Rural South Africa: An Innovative Approach*. Third edition. Amsterdam: VU University Press.

Vermeer, A., Wijnroks, L. & Magyarszeky, Z. (2008). Effects of Conductive Education in a Home for Children with Developmental Disabilities. In: Vermeer, A. & Tempelman, H.A. (Eds.), *Health Care in Rural South Africa: An Innovative Approach* (pp. 313-330). Third edition. Amsterdam: VU University Press.

Waal, M., de (2008). Turning the Tide: A Qualitative Study of ARV Treatment Programmes. In: Vermeer, A. & Tempelman, H.A. (Eds.), *Health Care in Rural South Africa: An Innovative Approach* (pp. 405-432). Third edition. Amsterdam: VU University Press.

With, A. de, Wouters, M. & Jongmans, M. (2008). Influences on the Nutritional Status of Children. In: Vermeer, A., & Tempelman, H.A. (Eds.), *Health Care in Rural South Africa: An Innovative Approach* (pp. 125-148). Third edition. Amsterdam: VU University Press.

Appendix 1: Guidelines for a Programme Research Proposal

These guidelines are derived from internationally accepted guidelines for submitting a research proposal or a plan for a research project. The application is particularly meant for the evaluation of the outcomes of a NCG programme. A research proposal according to international standards has to consist of the following elements:

1. **Preliminary title**
   - *as short as possible*
   - *eventually a subtitle (e.g. 'subject of the study': A literature review)*
2. **Introduction**
   - *motive for the research or background, e.g.*
     - derived from practice
     - derived from a relevant theory, application of a relevant theory
   - *aim of the research, e.g.*
     - to solve a practical problem
     - to gain insight into ......
     - to test an expectation/hypothesis
   - *type of research, e.g.*
     - literature study
     - descriptive study
     - explorative study
     - hypothesis testing
     - construction of a measuring instrument
     - intervention study
   - *indication of the target group*
   - *frame of reference (theoretical)*
   - *summary of earlier research*
   - *research questions or hypotheses*
   - *expected outcomes*
3. **Method**
   - *subjects/research group*
     - N men-women/boys-girls
     - age
     - level of development, e.g. IQ, grade at school
     - extent of the disease (progression)
     - phase of treatment or training
   - *measuring instruments/research methods*
     - e.g. test, observation, questionnaire, interview, focus group, Delphi method
     - reliability, e.g. test-retest, inter-/intra-observer reliability, internal consistency
     - validity, e.g., content, construct, concurrent, predictive
     - level of measurement: nominal, ordinal, interval/ratio
     - methods have to be related to each research question
   - *design*

- type of the study, e.g. quantitative or qualitative
- way of measuring/testing
- *statistics/methods of analysis, e.g.*
  - parametric/non-parametric
  - quantitative data processing: SPSS
  - qualitative data processing: WINMAX
- *procedure, e.g.*
  - how to engage the subjects
  - organizational aspects

4. **Phases of the research and time needed**
   - *literature study*
   - *introduction to the field of study*
   - *finding the subjects/research group*
   - *data collection*
   - *data processing*
   - *writing the research report/article*

5. **Requested budget**
   - *personnel*
   - *materials*
   - *travelling costs*
   - *gifts and honoraria*
   - *overhead costs*
   - *costs for the report or publication*

6. **Supervision**
   - *internal, e.g. within the organisation, or external, e.g. a university*
   - *participation in research meetings*
   - *intervision*

7. **Ethical aspects**
   - *informed consent*
   - *information to the subjects before and after*
   - *information about outcomes*

When the study is finished, a research report or a scientific article has to be written. Guidelines for this are:

8. **Results**
   - *overview of outcomes related to each research question*
   - *no comments, no conclusions*

9. **Conclusions and discussion**
   - *conclusions only based on outcomes*
   - *relationship between outcomes and earlier research or literature reports*
   - *contribution to the theory*
   - *constraints or problems during the research*
   - *expectations about the usefulness of the outcomes*
   - *alternative hypotheses*
   - *practical implications*
   - *recommendations for further research*

10. **References**
    - *style, e.g. APA (also for tables and figures)*
11. **Address of first author/Correspondence address**
12. **Appendices, e.g.**
    - *a new measuring instrument*
    - *a set of guidelines used*
13. **Abstract**
    - *native language and English*
    - *translate also the title of the report/article*
14. **Key words**

These guidelines form a set of 'ideal' guidelines. It will be obvious that the application of each element depends on the type of research to be carried out. When writing a research article for a scholarly journal, it is recommended to take an already published article as an example.

Chapter 6

Aspects of a Programme: How to Describe a Programme

Adri Vermeer[a]

Abstract

A frame of reference for programme description consists of the following aspects: introduction, describing the history and starting point of a programme; target group; aims; assessment of the starting position of the target group; working methods; evaluation; organisation; and research regarding the programme. By means of such a programme description it is possible to evaluate the content and the internal consistency of a programme and to compare similar programmes with each other.

1. Introduction

This chapter provides a frame of reference for the description of the programmes carried out under the umbrella of the Ndlovu Care Group (NCG). By means of these programmes NCG tries to realize its integrated care mission in rural areas of South Africa. It is the task of every professional care organization to make the translation of the mission into activities as transparent as possible. For an open interaction between care professionals and their clients, it has to be clear what kind of views on care and behavioural change are held by the professionals who try to change the lives and the behaviour of the people who participate in the programmes and who are subject to the programme's activities. The rationale for the care activities has to be evidence-based. This means that the theoretical or philosophical underpinnings are clearly described. And, if they are not yet clear or available because of the still explorative nature of a programme, personal views or naive starting points have to be expressed and written down. Next, professionally carried out care programmes need to be assessed by monitoring and evaluation procedures (see Chapter 4) and intervention research (see Chapter 5). Before such evaluation activities can be carried out, the aims and methods of a specific programme have to be clearly described. If it is not clear what kind of goals a programme is aiming at, it is not possible to determine and describe its outcomes. Intervention methods used in a specific programme have to be chosen on the basis of the expectation that a certain programme goal could be reached by the execution of the programme activities. If the relationship between a programme goal and a programme method is clearly described and theoretically un-

---

a. Professor emeritus of Special Education, Faculty of Social and Behavioural Sciences, Utrecht University, The Netherlands

derpinned, we call this aspect the *internal validity* of a programme. If it is established that a specific programme has proven results in a specific group of clients, and these results are also confirmed in a similar group at another place or another time, then we say that the programme has proven *external validity*.

This all means that a professional care organisation like NCG can provide a clear description of its programmes by using a frame of reference that consists of the following basic components or aspects:

starting points → target group → aims → methods → evaluation

We call this a *formal* frame of reference. It is 'formal' because it does not have a philosophical or theoretical content specifically chosen as a starting point for the programme to be described. This means that it is a theoretically or philosophically independent frame of reference. In other words, it is a kind of methodology for the description of programme contents.

Two formal frames of reference are used to describe the NCG programmes which form the contents of this book.

First, the organizational chart of NCG provides a descriptive model to give each programme its place within the organizational context of NCG (see Chapter 1). The organizational chart will be used to arrange the contents of this book into three parts.

Second, the frame of reference that will be used to describe the contents of each programme (see below). It is employed by the authors of the programme chapters of this book. It is derived from the literature which analyses the content of health care or educational programmes (e.g. Keith, 1984).

2. Frame of Reference for Programme Description

The frame of reference for the description of an NCG programme consists of a number of aspects. For each aspect, examples derived from NCG programmes will be given. The complete set of aspects provides an ideal description of a programme. It could be that a distinct aspect is not relevant for a specific programme or that a distinct aspect is not yet well elaborated, and it will be left out. The advantage of using such a frame of reference is that all programmes are described in the same way. This provides possibilities for comparison and content analysis.

2.1. Starting Points

A programme description usually starts with a short description of the *history* or the *course of development* of the programme. From this, the second aspect becomes evident: the *starting points* of the programme. This aspect tries to answer questions like:
- why the programme has been designed;
- why a specific programme has been chosen for a specific target population;
- why the programme is expected to result in the intended outcomes (see Chapter 4 and 5);
- why the programme could have the expected impact on the target population (see Chapter 4 and 5).

Various *classifications* provide the possibility to describe the goals and other aspects of a specific programme according to a relevant system. Examples include:
- the one described in this chapter: the function of this classification is to give distinct aspects of a programme a place in relationship to each other;
- the International Classification of Human Functioning (ICF): this classification describes the complex consequences of a disease or disorder for human functioning in terms of restricted activities of daily life and social participation (WHO, 2002);
- the Diagnostic Statistical Manual of Diseases: this classification sums up the characteristics of a specific disease or disorder (DSM IV-TR, 2004);
- the Millennium Development Goals for South Africa (UNO, 2007): this classification allows NCG to relate its general goals to a national/international framework for solving the world's main developmental challenges.

It is characteristic of classifications that there are no proven relationships (e.g. causal) between the distinct aspects of the classification.

Starting points can be divided into:
- *Philosophical starting points*: they describe views on human existence or societal functioning. An example is the NCG mission for their work in the rural areas where NCG is active (see Chapter 1). A characteristic of these kinds of starting points is that relationships between distinct aspects of the specific starting point cannot be proved by empirical research. The relationships are based on views. The function of philosophical starting points is to elucidate/support the choice for the development of specific programmes to improve the living in a specific socio-economic context and the choice for specific theoretical models for the validation of these programmes.
- *Theoretical starting points*: these kinds of starting points describe empirically verified relationships between the aspects of a specific theoretical model. An example is NCG research carried out to establish the expected outcomes of the NNU (see Chapter 12) or the NAAP programme (see Chapter 12) by using the Ajzen (1991) theory of changing social behaviour. The function of a theoretical model here is to explain why a programme could expect specific outcomes.

Chosen starting points have to be translated or adapted to be used as an underpinning for a specific NCG programme. For example, if the ICF is used to describe the complex consequences of HIV/AIDS, the following characteristics could be derived from the definition of its three main components, namely:
1. physiological and neurological *dysfunctions* caused by HIV infection and AIDS;
2. restricted *activities* as a consequence of the physiological or anatomical disorder, e.g. restrictions in the execution of daily activities and learning activities;
3. restricted social *participation* as a consequence of the restriction of activities, e.g. restrictions in family interaction, visiting school, and participation in work.

This kind of classification is helpful to assess the complex consequences of HIV/AIDS. It is also helpful to indicate which consequence of the disease has to become the focus of the treatment. For example, AntiRetroViral's concern the treatment of the physiological consequences. Thereafter, the focus has to be on learning to cope with any persistent hindrances to carrying out activities of daily living. In the next phase of the treatment, attention has to be paid to the way the person with HIV/ AIDS could nevertheless learn to participate in social contexts, according to his/her capacities.

Clearly formulated starting points are not always present at the start of a programme. Mostly, there are views or vague concepts in the minds of the initiators. During the further development of the programme, these views and concepts become more and more concrete, and even a theoretical underpinning for the programme can be found.

2.2. Target Group or Target Population

The next aspect concerns the justification of the choice for a specific target group, e.g.:
- children, youth, parents;
- schoolchildren, farmers, mine workers;
- malnourished children, vulnerable children;
- other groups.

The identification of a specific target group for a specific programme implies the development of inclusion criteria for that programme. For example, when the Nutritional Unit Programme started, it aimed at malnourished and undernourished children. To be included in the programme, criteria for weight of the children in relation to age were formulated.

When the programme concerns a large group of people living in a certain area of a country, we can speak of a target population.

2.3. Aims

The central aspect of a programme concerns its aims. No clearly formulated aims means no possibility to monitor and evaluate a programme. Aims have the function to direct programme activities. If a programme activity could not be considered as a solid operationalisation of a programme aim, or the programme activity does not fit the aim, there is no internal consistency within the programme. It often happens that the aims of a programme are too general or too vague. Such a programme runs the risk of not being able to use such an aim as an internal criterion for the justification of specific programme activities.

We can discern between several kinds of aims:
a. *General aims:* these are final aims of a programme, in other words, long-term aims.
b. *Intermediary or temporary aims:* these are aims which could be achieved in a concrete situation and within a certain amount of time, in other words short-term aims.
c. *Concrete aims:* examples are aims for one client, or aims for a specific group, or aims per session or per week.

2.4 Assessment of the Starting Position of the Target Group/Population

Before a programme can start, insight has to be gained into the needs and desires, general health status, health status with regard to a specific disease, or developmental problems, or the specific behaviour to be changed; they have to be inventorised. Also, statistical baselines have to be established. Otherwise, the scale at which a specific programme has to be designed is not clear.

In the case of a target population, e.g. the population of Limpopo Province, epidemiological figures have to be collected. The support of national or regional governmental bodies is then needed. In case of a specific target group, e.g. schoolchildren in the Moutse area, smaller surveys could be carried out by the care organisation, mostly a NGO.

At the *real start* of the programme, the state of the disease, the level of functioning, the type and state of specific behaviour to be changed have to be assessed. To this end, diagnostic measurements could be used, or measuring instruments for programme evaluation. The former are used for admission to a programme: a person responds 'yes' or 'no' to the selection criterion. Evaluation measurements are designed to measure intra- and inter-individual differences or changes.

2.5. Working Methods

The working methods of a programme primarily concern the programme activities to be carried out. We can discern the following aspects:
a. *The content of the programme:* e.g. how information about the programme will be given and to whom; which teaching methods and which methods aiming at change will be used; which evaluation methods will be carried out; is there any kind of follow-up?
b. *Strategy, didactic plan/method*: what kind of interaction between professional(s) and clients will be used, e.g. information processing, confrontation, group discussions, changing behaviour methods like 'unfreezing, freezing, unfreezing'?
c. *Means:* practical issues like frequency of an activity, duration of the programme, use of video, teacher or parent involvement, use of experts, etc.

2.6. Evaluation

One feature of a professionally designed programme is that it has to be evaluated. Evaluation procedures can consist of M&E (see Chapter 4) and evidence-based research (see Chapter 5). Both focus on the assessing the internal and external validity of a programme.

Evaluation procedures have to be carried out at several timepoints during the execution of the programme:
1. *At the start of the programme:* see section 2.4, in particular measurement of e.g. the health or developmental status or behavioural status (= baseline).
2. *During the programme:* e.g. registration of the activities, presence of the participants, establishment of intermediate/temporary aims (= process evaluation), interim measurement of the health, developmental or behavioural effects.

3. *At the end of the programme:* establishment of the final effects of the programme (= product evaluation); evaluation of all procedural aspects and inventarisation of constraints (= process evaluation and M&E).
4. *After the end of the programme, also named 'follow-up':* is there continuity of outcomes, in other words, long-term effects; what is the impact of the programme on the lives of the clients or the community?

2.7. Organisation

Professional health care, developmental and educational programmes carried out by an NGO like NCG are developed and active in several environmental contexts. They can be geographic, organisational and political contexts. For a proper understanding of the possible impact of a programme, it is valuable to describe the relationships between the NGO responsible for the specific programme and the external bodies with which co-operation is necessary or desired. Embedment of the programme of an NGO like NCG in a broader context also contributes to the external validity of the programme. Kinds of external contexts include:
- relationship with similar kinds of programmes in the neighbourhood;
- co-operation with regional or national bodies;
- involvement of external expertise;
- international cooperation.

2.8. NCG Research

In this chapter, it has been stressed that research to establish the basis for a programme, also known as 'evidence-based research', has be to an integral part of the programme design and evaluation procedures of an NGO like NCG. Evidence-based research serves several purposes: to show the validity of the programmes to external bodies (e.g. sponsors and financiers); to validate implementation elsewhere; to improve the training of professionals for a specific programme inside and outside one's own NGO; to publish nationally and internationally about the outcomes and determinants of a programme. Therefore, it also has to be an integral part of a programme description to refer to research carried out to evaluate a specific programme.

3. Conclusion

This chapter provided a formal frame of reference for the description of the NCG programmes described in Parts Two and Three of this book. The purpose of this frame of reference is twofold.

First, its aim is to assist the managers of an NCG programme to reflect on whether programme activities are in accordance with the intended goals. If a relationship between a programme goal and a programme activity is not supported, we have to conclude that the internal validity of a specific programme is weak. That does not mean that a programme activity does not make sense. The only underpinning then is that the usefulness of a specific programme is based on experience. That is not a sufficient justification for the further implementation of a programme. The 'external world' would like to know the rationale behind a programme. In other words, what are the pretentions of a specific programme, or what kind of improvement, development or change a programme is aiming at.

Second, the use of the provided frame of reference allows programmes to be compared. This implies that comparable programmes have comparable outcomes. If the outcomes of comparable programmes differ, it is important to ascertain whether these differences are related to differences in the content of a programme, that is, to the discerned aspects of a programme.

References

Ajzen, I. (1991). The Theory of Planned Behaviour. *Organizational Behaviour and Human Decision Processes, 50,* 179-211.

Keith, R.A. (1984). Functional Assessment in Program Evaluation for Rehabilitation Medicine. In: Granger, C.V. & Gresham, G.E. (Eds.), *Functional Assessment in Rehabilitation Medicine* (pp. 122-139). Baltimore/London: Williams & Wilkins.

DSM IV-TR (2004). *Diagnostic and Statistical Manual of Mental Disorders, Text Revision IV.* Arlington, VA (USA): American Psychiatric Association.

UNO (2007). *The Millennium Development Goals Report 2007.* New York: United Nations.

WHO (2002). *International Classification of Functioning, Disability and Health (ICF).* Geneva: WHO.

Part Two

Clinical Services, the Autonomous Treatment Centre (ATC)

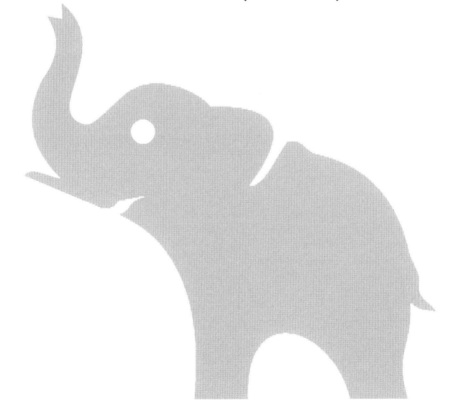

Chapter 7

The Autonomous Treatment Centre (ATC)

Hugo Tempelman[a,b], *Peter Schrooders*[c], *Mariette Slabbert*[d]

"A historic commitment to wellness initiatives will keep millions of Americans from setting foot in the doctor's office in the first place, because these are preventable diseases and we're going to invest in prevention."
President Obama (2 February 2009)

Abstract

The Autonomous Treatment Centre (ATC) is a rural 'one-stop shop' for integrated primary health services, including TB/HIV/AIDS, malaria, chronic disease management, and reproductive health at a community level. An ATC consists of a 12-hour clinic, a 24-hour clinic and support & diagnostic services. The decentralised clinical services supported by high-end technology guarantee accurate diagnosis and follow-up in underserved communities. The dedicated HIV monitoring laboratory and the radiology department change the face of resource-poor health care delivery. Accurate laboratory monitoring further facilitates task shifting, the delegation of tasks to the lowest level of personnel qualified to do the job, and enables the delivery of decentralised community health services. The ATC programmes are designed and measured at the primary, secondary, tertiary prevention, and retention through motivation levels, in the Rural Advancement Plan continuum of care.

1. Introduction

The Report of the Commission on Macro-economics and Health as well as the subsequent WHO report, *Scaling up the Response to Infectious Disease: A Way out of Poverty*, documented the incontrovertible links between health and economic development, and the rising health care demands related to infectious diseases such as HIV/AIDS and tuberculosis. More generally, the management of all chronic conditions – non-communicable diseases, long-term mental disorders, and certain communicable diseases such as HIV/AIDS – is one of the greatest challenges facing health care systems throughout the world. Currently, chronic conditions are responsible for 60% of the global disease burden. They are increasing such that by the year

---

a. CEO Ndlovu Care Group, Groblersdal, South Africa
b. Visiting Professor, Faculty of Social and Behavioural Sciences, Faculty of Medicine, Utrecht University, The Netherlands
c. Medical Director Ndlovu Medical Centre, Elandsdoorn, South Africa
d. COO Ndlovu Care Group, Groblersdal, South Africa

2020, developing countries can expect 80% of their disease burden to come from chronic problems. In these countries, adherence to therapies is as low as 20%, resulting in poor health outcomes at a very high cost to society, governments, and families.

The Alma Ata Declaration on Primary Health Care (WHO-UNICEF, 1978) defines primary health care as "essential health care based on practical, scientifically sound and socially acceptable methods and technology, made universally accessible to individuals and families in the community through their full participation and at a cost that the community and the country can afford to maintain at every stage of their development in the spirit of self-reliance and self-determination".

According to the University of Cape Town, Faculty of Health Sciences,[1] primary health care (PHC) is therefore understood as an approach to health care that promotes the attainment by all people of a level of health that will permit them to live socially and economically productive lives. PHC is health care that is essential, scientifically sound (evidence-based), ethical, accessible, equitable, affordable, and accountable to the community. In other words, PHC is not just primary medical or curative care, nor is it a package of low-cost medical interventions for the poor and marginalised. On the contrary, it calls for the integration of health services in the process of community development, a process that requires political commitment, intersectoral collaboration, and multidisciplinary involvement for success.

In a 2002 speech to the Commonwealth Club in San Francisco, Gloria Steinem observed, "We are still standing on the bank of the river, rescuing people who are drowning. We have not gone to the head of the river to keep them from falling in. That is the 21st century task." Steinem's remark refers to a popular analogy, 'Moving Upstream', that is used to highlight the importance and relevance of primary prevention (Ardell, 1977/1986; in: Cohen, Chávez, & Chehimi, 2007; p.4). 'Moving Upstream' is described as follows: "While walking along the banks of a river, a passerby notices that someone in the water is drowning. After pulling the person ashore, the rescuer notices another person in the river in need of help. Before long, the river is filled with drowning people, and more rescuers are required to assist the initial rescuer. Unfortunately, some people are not saved, and some victims fall back into the river after they have been pulled ashore. At this time, one of the rescuers starts walking upstream. 'Where are you going?' the other rescuers ask, disconcerted. The upstream rescuer replies, 'I'm going upstream to see why so many people keep falling into the river.' As it turns out, the bridge leading across the river upstream has a hole through which people are falling." The upstream rescuer realizes that fixing the hole in the bridge will prevent many people from ever falling into the river in the first place. The act of 'moving upstream' and taking action *before* a problem arises in order to avoid it entirely, rather than treating or alleviating its consequences, is called primary prevention.

The term *primary prevention* was coined in the late 1940s by Leavell and Clark from the Harvard and Columbia University Schools of Public Health, respectively. Leavell and Clark described primary prevention as "measures applicable to a particular disease or group of diseases in order to intercept the causes of disease before they involve man . . . [in the form of] specific immunizations, attention to personal hygiene, use of environmental sanitation, protection against occupational hazards, protection from accidents, use of specific nutrients, protection from carcinogens, and avoidance of allergens" (in: Morgan & Goldston, 1987; p. 3). Although Leavell and Clark's definition is mostly disease-oriented, the applications of primary prevention extend beyond medical problems and include the prevention of other societal concerns, ranging from violence to environmental degradation, that also affect health and well-being. Primary prevention efforts are proactive, by definition, and should generally be aimed at populations, not just individuals. Returning to the upstream analogy, fixing the hole in the bridge will benefit not only those at greatest risk for falling in but everyone who crosses it, the rescuers on the riverbank, and everyone who helps pay for rescue costs.

Leavell and Clark further identified two other degrees of prevention, termed *secondary* and *tertiary prevention*. Secondary prevention consists of a set of measures used for early detection and prompt intervention to control a problem or disease and minimize the consequences, while tertiary prevention focuses on the reduction of further complications of an existing disease or problem, through treatment and rehabilitation (Spasoff, Harris, & Thuriaux, 2001). Leavell and Clark's 'overarching concept of prevention' actually refers to three distinct activities that might be better termed 'prevention, treatment, and rehabilitation' (Morgan & Goldston, 1987; p. 3). As noted by Albee (1987; in: Cohen et al., 2007), "All three forms of preventive intervention are useful and defensible". While primary prevention *alone* is not enough to address pervasive health and social problems, it remains the foremost method that we can employ in order to *eliminate* future health and social problems. Albee goes on to note that "any *reduction in incidence* must rely heavily on proactive efforts with large groups, and such actions involve primary prevention approaches" (see also Chapter 9).

During the CDC's 2003 National HIV Prevention Conference in Atlanta (USA), Mary Linn Hemphill pointed out: "If we are serious about improving the health and quality of life of Americans *and* keeping our health care budget under control . . . we cannot afford to ignore the power of prevention" (p. 6 of the Conference Introduction). Health care is among the most expensive commitments of government, businesses, and individuals combined. A targeted investment in prevention not only decreases the financial burden on the health care system but also staves off unnecessary and rising medical costs. According to the US Preventive Services Task Forces' *Guide to Clinical Preventive Services* (1996), primary prevention is generally considered the most cost-effective way to provide effective health care, due to its role in alleviating the unnecessary suffering and high costs of specialized care associated with disease. A primary prevention approach also helps defer the social costs associated with illness and injury that arise from lost productivity and expenditures for disability, workers' compensation, and public benefit programmes.

2. Health Care Service

NCG, through the Rural Advancement Plan (RAP), wants to apply its model of prevention and motivation to strengthen health care delivery through the ATC in South Africa. Assisting the Department of Health in strengthening the District Health Services is an enormous challenge for NGOs. In the past, even reaching a dialogue around cooperation was difficult to achieve. It was Barbara Hogan, Minister for

Health of South Africa, who opened the dialogue with NGOs and created a vision of public-private partnerships during her short term in office in 2008. The *Pocket Guide to District Health Care in SA²* (Harrison in Health Systems Trust, 1997) defines a district health system as the vehicle for providing quality primary health care to everyone in a defined geographical area. It is a system of health care in which individuals, communities, and all the health care providers of the area participate together in improving their own health. The pocket guide identifies[3] five important characteristics of district-based PHC.

2.1. The Service Responds to Health Needs

A good district-based primary health care service will be organised to respond, first and foremost, to the greatest need. For example, if tuberculosis is a leading cause of death and disease, services must be geared to deal effectively with TB. This means that we need a clear understanding of the major health problems in our districts, and a way of deciding whether our actions are making any difference. Because money always seems to be in short supply, we need to organise our services so that we give the greatest priority to the greatest problems.

2.2. The Service Views People as a Whole

Imagine taking a car along to the garage on a Monday to have it serviced and the radiator fixed, only to be told that the service will be done today, but that the day for fixing radiators is only Thursdays! It sounds funny, but that's the way we have run our health service. A child with a minor ailment might be seen on a Monday, treated and told to return to the child health clinic on Wednesday because she is overdue for immunisations. Worse still, she may be told to go to the local authority clinic because "they do the vaccinations". We need to bring our services together into a "one-stop shop" so that people are treated as a whole and not like body parts!

Re-organisation of Services

This is going to mean quite a lot of *re-organisation of our services*. First, local authority and provincial clinics will both need to offer the full range of services, instead of local authorities focussing on prevention and provincial clinics on treatment. Many nurses will need to brush up on their skills and knowledge and may require further training. Second, we need to move away from services organised so that when children come on Mondays, antenatal care is provided on Tuesdays, immunisations on Wednesdays, and family planning on Thursdays. People should be able to get the service they need on any day.

Integrated PHC Programmes

PHC *programmes* such as maternal and child health, nutrition and oral health are activities which will improve each aspect of health, but it does *not* mean that each programme will be run separately. For example, if you are a nurse attending to a two-year-old child, you will be concerned with all three aspects of the child's health mentioned here. By identifying specific PHC programmes, we ensure that all aspects of health care receive attention, and that you as a frontline health worker are helped to implement the programme activities as part of your daily work.

The Patient as a Person

As health workers, we often have to deal with some of the most basic of human sensations, like pain and discomfort. People come to you to seek help and relief from these experiences. In their eyes, feeling cared for and being treated with *dignity* are probably the most important measures of the quality of their care. One way of showing respect is to allow patients to become active participants in their own health care. This is done by sharing the appropriate amount of information with them during the healing process. Another important aspect is *confidentiality*, as people's right to privacy is an important part of their self-esteem and total well-being.

2.3. The Service Is Concerned with People's Health, Not Just Disease

A good PHC service is concerned with the health of all of the people in the district, not just with treating disease. In other words, the service is comprised of five aspects, namely:
– promotion of good health;
– prevention of disease and trauma;
– cure of illness;
– rehabilitation;
– palliation (when required).

Promotion of Good Health

The district health team needs to decide *what* the most important health messages are which they want to convey, and *how* they are going to get those messages across. Giving 'general health education' to people in packed waiting rooms is often not the best way to get important messages to people. We need to develop a health promotion strategy for each district. We do this by deciding on:
– the most important health problems in our district;
– key health promotion messages for each health problem;
– strategies for getting these messages across.

For example, you may determine that diarrhoeal disease is a major problem. You may then decide that the key message you want people to hear is that they should use clean water (boiled or with *chlorinated bleach* added). You should then decide on strategies for getting this message across, such as discussions in women's groups or churches.

Infection with HIV and AIDS will be a priority in every district. After you decide which messages you are using, they should become the *consistent* messages throughout the district. You will need to decide on strategies for getting these messages across, such as school discussions, drama presentations, and convincing church leaders to help get the message across.

Prevention of Disease and Trauma

Your efforts at prevention must be geared to addressing the biggest preventable problems. If you identify child and woman abuse, high blood pressure and car accidents as three priority problems which can be prevented, you need to develop strategies for prevention around each of them. These strategies may need to be developed jointly with other sectors like the Departments of Welfare or Transport, and with NGOs. For example, your efforts to prevent *abuse of children and women* may focus on a district awareness campaign in collaboration with local community-based organisations and Child Welfare. You may also set up a system of early referral for children whom you or schoolteachers suspect may be being abused.

Strategies to prevent *high blood pressure* or its complications may focus on promoting good eating habits, early diagnosis through routine screening, and proper management of hypertensive patients. You may work closely with the Department of Transport to prevent *car accidents*. Together, you may initiate a community campaign to promote better road safety, reduce drunk driving, and erect proper railings along roads frequently used by children walking to school.

Cure of Illness

The curative part of health cure takes the largest share of the budget, so it is important that treatment is only given when really needed, and that the cheapest effective treatment is given. We need to improve the *prescribing habits* of both doctors and nurses to reduce the number of medicines given, and to ensure that the medicines given are appropriate. Some of the biggest problems at the moment are:
– over-prescription of antibiotics;
– handing out too many medicines;
– poor explanation to patients of what their problems are, and how to take the medicines.

All health workers involved in clinical care need to continue to *update their knowledge* and skills, so that they provide the best cost-effective service possible. One of the responsibilities of the district management team is to ensure that there are opportunities for continuing medical education and getting information.

Rehabilitation

South Africa should be especially concerned about rehabilitation. The violence of our society has left many people emotionally, psychologically and physically scarred. Inadequate and ineffective occupational safety regulations have meant that many workers have been injured or debilitated in some way, and left without adequate support or rehabilitation. Alcohol and drug abuse are big problems in many communities. But rehabilitation has been a very neglected part of health care. Each district needs to

develop strategies for each aspect of rehabilitation, physical, mental or psychological. And the capacity of each district to provide rehabilitation needs to be built up by:
- enabling health workers to recognise people requiring rehabilitation;
- ensuring that there are appropriate rehabilitation workers in the district;
- creating referral links between the health services, NGOs and other sectors;
- encouraging community-based rehabilitation.

Health workers need to be trained to *recognise problems* which require treatment and rehabilitation. This is particularly true of mental and psychological problems, where a high proportion of people receive no therapy and rehabilitative support. At the moment, very few districts have occupational therapists or physiotherapists, for example. Where they are present, they either work exclusively in the private sector or only see hospital patients. Because of the shortage of these types of health workers, we need to use every one of them to the benefit of the entire district community. This will mean a rethink of the role of hospital-based therapists and developing ways in which private sector professionals can become involved in rehabilitation strategies *for the whole district*. In many instances, the only community-based rehabilitation services are being provided by NGOs. We need to create good *referral mechanisms* between the public health sector and NGOs, as well as to other departments like welfare. We should also find ways in which we can continue to reach people requiring rehabilitation even once they have left hospital and returned home. In some areas of South Africa, community-based rehabilitation workers have proved to be a cost-effective way of providing community outreach and follow-up.

Palliation

Palliation means to remove pain and discomfort. We usually use this term when we speak of managing patients who cannot be cured, or who are going to die. Previously, we glossed over this aspect of PHC, but as more and more people die of AIDS, we need to be able to relieve pain and discomfort for people dying at home.

2.4. *The Service Also Includes District Hospital Care*

District-based health care includes those services provided by the district (level 1) hospital. In practice, this means health care which a general medical practitioner can reasonably be expected to provide. This should include:
- basic surgery, like circumcisions, appendectomies, and most trauma emergencies;
- obstetric care, like assisted vaginal deliveries and Caesarian sections;
- basic anaesthetics;
- setting of fractures;
- other basic surgical, medical and diagnostic procedures.

District hospital services must be regarded as part of the provision of comprehensive PHC, because they form the first level of support and referral for primary care. Unless level 1 hospital services are seen as part of the district health system, we will create a divide between clinic or community-based care and hospital care. One of the problems which districts will need to overcome is the fact that most hospitals are, in effect, managed by the Medical Superintendent, Hospital Administrator and Nursing Services Manager, while clinics now fall under the district management team. The district hospital cannot operate in isolation and will need to become part of the district health service.

2.5. The Service Has Clear Systems of Referral

An important part of clinical care within districts is a proper *referral system*. This referral system must ensure that:
– sick people are treated by appropriately trained personnel;
– frontline health workers have support and back-up for decision making.

Most of the clinics within our districts are staffed by nursing clinical practitioners, and not by doctors. Some health centres may have general practitioners to whom people may be referred, but in many cases a sick person (or some one needing further investigation) may need to be referred straight to the district hospital. But the referral system within the district must not end there! The referring practitioner needs to be informed of the outcome of the referral and often needs to be informed of continuing follow-up of the patient following discharge.

But the other aspect of a referral system that is very much neglected in South Africa is a way in which health workers can consult other colleagues and seek advice. Often, the patient does not need referral from the clinic to hospital, or from one hospital to another, the practitioner attending the patient just wants advice! This can be done by phone or fax, but electronic communication should make this type of referral much easier.

President Zuma acknowledged this in his State of the Nation Address during the opening of Parliament, June 2009: *"We have set ourselves the goals of further reducing inequalities in health care provision, to boost human resource capacity, revitalize hospitals and clinics and step up the fight against the scourge of HIV and AIDS, tuberculosis and other diseases. We must work together to improve the implementation of the Comprehensive Plan for the Treatment, Management and Care of HIV and AIDS so as to reduce the rate of new HIV infections by 50% by the year 2011. We want to reach 80% of those in need of ARV treatment also by 2011. We will introduce a National Health Insurance (NHI) scheme in a phased and incremental manner. In order to initiate the NHI, the urgent rehabilitation of public hospitals will be undertaken through Public-Private Partnerships."*[4]

3. Ndlovu Care Group's Clinical Care

Over the years, NCG has developed and standardised a quality clinical care and treatment centre that decentralises the provision of integrated health care to the community level. The motivation for total decentralisation of services lies in the difficulty in delivering services in rural areas: lack of infrastructure, logistical chain management, and bringing care to the client's doorstep. In a country like South Africa that is so severely struck by the double epidemic of TB and HIV/AIDS, only a strong, decentralised District Health Care system can provide essential services to the underserved rural areas. NGOs should not try to replace the government's responsibility for public service delivery but should rather contribute with innovative methods, support with building service capacity and delivery, and assistance with the implementation of government programmes. Responsible NGOs do not duplicate through parallel systems but develop sustainable support for public service delivery.

In South Africa, the controversial stance of the government around HIV/AIDS management over the last few years created an opportunity for direct donor funding to NGOs. With new leadership, the time is ripe to integrate these services and invest actively in public-private partnerships (PPPs) to support the reconstruction of a strong Public Health Care Service delivery system. NGOs need to invest in relationships with the Department of Health at all levels, to create an environment where the assistance of NGOs and private institutions is seen in the positive role of contributors, rather than as a threat or competition.

The donors could act as the brokers that harmonise the integration of NGOs into the public system to add extra capacity in under-resourced areas.

NCG wants to establish strategic PPPs with the relevant government departments, institutional donors (e.g. USAID/PEPFAR, BM Gates Foundation, Netherlands Embassy, DFID, etc), corporations through their social corporate responsibility programmes, and private investors. These PPPs render the comprehensive NCG Rural Advancement Plan (Community Health & Community Care services) sustainable within the framework and policies of the government's plans. NCG would like to penetrate more rural areas through similar PPPs to assist the government with its integrated, sustainable, rural development strategy. This chapter describes the Autonomous Treatment Centre and all its components and its functions.

It is NCG's vision and mission to align its tasks within the framework of the Millennium Development Goals (MDGs) defined by the United Nations, the HIV & AIDS and STI Strategic Plan for South Africa 2007-2011 (NSP 2007-2011), the national strategic plans of other departments (Education, Arts & Culture, etc.) and the Three Ones Strategy defined by the major donor organisations (as explained in Chapter 1). Through the ATC, the NCG contributes to the following MDGs:
- Promote gender equality & empower women
- Reduce child mortality
- Improve maternal health
- Combat HIV/AIDS, malaria, etc.

4. The Autonomous Treatment Centre

The ATC provides holistic community health services, with the emphasis on integrated quality of PHC, which includes chronic disease management, TB and HIV/AIDS, reproductive health, inpatient care, and support services. The ATC is a community-based centre of excellence, and as such, it addresses several of South Africa's major problems, namely:
- remigration and attraction of scarce skills to rural areas;
- the creation of capacity (through skills development) and employment through comprehensive health delivery;

- addressing HIV/AIDS and TB by providing outpatient and inpatient care in the areas where the epidemic is at its worst, viz. the rural areas;
- delegating responsibility for community health back to the community where it occurs.

One of the differentiating aspects of service delivery of the NCG Rural Advancement Plan is that all programmes, including ATC, are designed and measured through the same *continuum of care*. The NCG RAP continuum of care includes primary, secondary, tertiary prevention and retention (through motivation).

Prevention outcomes are tracked across prevention and motivation interventions to ensure that means are not confused with ends or, to put it differently, that outputs are not confused with outcomes (see Chapter 4):

- *Primary prevention*: All attempts are aimed at curbing seroconversion and detecting HIV occurrence early in the population. This is achieved through the 'Go MAD' strategy that promotes mobilisation, awareness, and destigmatisation. The measurement of primary prevention is the number of individuals targeted for counselling, and the percentage of the target group that agrees to undergo Voluntary Counselling and Testing (VCT+). This means that VCT+ is counted as an entry point into care and not as an end in itself.
- *Secondary prevention*: People who test positive during the primary prevention stage are followed up with a CD4 count, TB screening and counselling session, to stage the progress of HIV. This enables staff to provide the patients who test positive with a treatment plan and estimated timelines of interventions, e.g. when antiretroviral treatment (ART) will be started, etc. Six-monthly CD4 and viral load testing continues for life. The objective of secondary prevention is to convince HIV+ clients to seek health care early when they experience signs and symptoms and to remain in the monitoring programme. The measurement of secondary prevention is the percentage of individuals who tested positive during VCT+, undergo CD4, are screened for TB, and are provided with a treatment plan.
- *Tertiary prevention*: When HIV progresses and the CD4 falls to around 350, the clients are initiated on lifelong ART. Early initiation prevents morbidity and mortality and ensures that clients can lead a healthy life. Measurements for tertiary prevention include the percentage of patients attending their ATC appointments.
- *Retention*: Once clients are enrolled in RAP programmes, they have to attend motivation programmes to promote adherence to treatment. With clients on ART, the objective is adherence above 95%. Adherence is a real challenge as clients are not allowed to miss more that three doses in a month. Measurements of retention include the percentage of patients following their treatment plans, including six-monthly monitoring.

The ATC has four legs, namely (1) the 12-hour Community Health Centre, (2) the 24-hour Maternity and Inpatient Clinic, (3) the Counselling Service, and (4) the Decentralised Laboratory, X-ray, Pharmaceutical and M&E Services.

4.1. The 12-Hour Community Health Centre

The Ndlovu Care Group's 12-hour Community Health Centre (CHC) not only reaches out and provides health care to rural communities, but also empowers these communities to take responsibility for their own health, through cross-referral among all the programmes that fit under the RAP umbrella. Collectively, the programmes address the holistic continuum of care that includes primary, secondary, and tertiary prevention of chronic, acute and infectious diseases, including HIV & AIDS and TB. VCT+ plays a major role as an entry point into the RAP strategy in community work as well as in the clinic services. In the RAP model, everybody should know his/her HIV status, and each contact with the community serves as an opportunity to offer a VCT. On the ATC side, PHC and the TB programme are opportunities to increase VCT+ uptake. For the prevention strategy that underpins the RAP model, it is essential to detect disease early. VCT+ refers to HIV counselling and testing that are immediately followed up by a CD4 count, to stage positive individuals at the time of testing, and TB questionnaire screening. Performing a CD4 count at the time of diagnosis enables the caregiver to present these clients with an individual referral, treatment, and care plan. Women are offered a PAP smear as a cervical cancer screening method as well.

The 12-hour CHC addresses prevention at all three levels by screening and staging for early detection, controlling existing diseases through monitoring, caring and treating to promote early care-seeking behaviour, and preventing morbidity and mortality. The CHC motivates adherence and compliance to treatment regimens through intensive counselling and defaulter tracing. Intensive counselling establishes patient confidence in the clinical services, and it improves patient adherence, patient compliance, and patient retention in NCG programmes. NCG achieves considerable economies of scale, skills development, and accesses a large numbers of clients with this holistic prevention approach,.

4.2. The 24-Hour Clinic (Maternity and Inpatient Care)

The Ndlovu Care Group recognises that certain health issues cannot be managed in a 'quick-in/quick-out' manner, and thus established its 24-hour clinic. This clinic provides services for:
1. Reproductive health, maternal and neonatal care: community-based family planning, antenatal care and obstetrics with postnatal follow-up programmes.
2. PMTCT programme for HIV+ pregnant women.
3. TB/HIV & AIDS inpatient care supports patients from the TB and HAART programmes who cannot be managed on an outpatient level. In the RAP model, the last group of patients is managed in care centres at the community level instead of district hospitals, where family members can assist with non-clinical functions. The current capacity in the hospitals cannot provide the intensive nursing, support, and nutritional care these patients require. The ATC clinical staff provides the necessary medical care, while the family assists with nutritional and support care.

4.3. Counselling Service

The importance of good counselling is emphasized by the fact that adherence is delegated to individuals with no previous training in psychology or health care. In line with the RAP principle of skills development of the local community, and employment from the community, NCG offers local recruits intensive adherence counselling training programmes.

Counsellors in RAP perform both VCT+ and adherence counselling. VCT+ plays a major role as an entry point into the RAP strategy in community work as well as in the clinical services. As NCG believes that everybody should know his/her HIV status, each contact with the clinic serves as an opportunity to offer a VCT. PHC and the TB programme are vehicles for VCT+ uptake and early detection of HIV.

VCT+ refers to counselling and testing that are immediately followed up by a CD4 count, TB questionnaire screening, and staging to present these clients with an individual referral, treatment, and care plan. The individual treatment plan establishes patient confidence in the clinical service and improves patient adherence, patient compliance, and patient retention in NCG programmes. At the ATC, women are offered a PAP smear as a cervical cancer screening method, and they are referred for colposcopy if necessary. Because adherence to ART is vital, NCG invests a lot of effort in ensuring that the counselling at its facilities is of a high standard. Counsellors who perform counselling services are trained both in-service and through external training programmes. They are also continuously evaluated and retrained when necessary. Career development for counsellors acts as a motivator together with debriefing to ensure counsellor welfare and confidence.

Adherence counselling topics cover every aspect of counselling, ranging from chronic diseases, HIV & AIDS, TB, social, cultural, and psychological aspects. Counselling sessions are standardised, and counsellors use flipcharts and tick sheets to ensure that all topics are covered in each patient session and that the messages are delivered consistently. Clients who report to the clinic are screened and counselled at every visit, and counsellors are trained to observe and prompt clients to determine when they need referral to other services. Clients who fail to report for their appointments are traced and re-introduced to the programmes after the reason for defaulting is established and addressed. Counsellors are the frontline employees for client contact and need to act and perform in a professional manner. In this light, NCG recognises its counsellors as valued members of the professional team that flags patient complaints and underlying disease.

4.4. Decentralised Diagnostic and Support Services

These diagnostic and support services enable the operation of the ATCs and make the ATCs relatively independent of service delivery. The isolation and lack of infrastructure in most rural areas makes it impractical and often impossible to transfer blood and pathology samples and to refer patients for further diagnosis and treatment. In the absence of public transport, radiology facilities for instance are out of reach for most rural communities. The following enabling services create the management environment needed to govern the ATC at a local level.

HIV Monitoring Laboratory for Local HIV/AIDS Management

HIV is easily and accurately monitored through viral load, CD4 count, full blood count, and blood chemistry. These values provide a demarcated framework for laboratory testing and indicate the effect of treatment interventions. Through volume-driven systems and systemic processes, NCG reduces the cost and utilises human resources to a maximum extent. One peripheral HIV monitoring laboratory can serve approximately 15,000 patients on ART with a staff equivalent of two laboratory technicians, an administrative person, and a data capturer. Through IT infrastructure, the daily results are e-mailed to and signed off by a pathologist, in line with the rules and regulations of the National Health Act. The peripheral laboratories are SANAC accredited.

X-ray and Ultrasound Facilities

Digital X-ray facilities assist with the detection of TB and the management of injuries. Digitalisation necessitates a higher initial investment, but the benefits far outweigh conventional radiology in rural settings. Images can be taken, immediately examined, deleted, corrected, and subsequently sent to a network of computers. Digital radiology makes the facility filmless. The referring physician can view the requested image on a desktop personal computer, often with the report, just minutes after the examination was performed. The images are no longer held in a single location; they can be seen simultaneously by different physicians and can be e-mailed for second opinions. In addition, the facility does not need a darkroom, it saves on developing consumables and storage space, and the patient can have all his or her X-rays on a CD to take to another physician or hospital.

Sonar Equipment

Sonar equipment supports the 24-hour unit in monitoring pregnant women to detect the duration of pregnancy (dating the pregnancy), uncover fetal abnormalities and monitor fetal development and growth.

Colposcopy and LLETZ Laser

The colposcopy system uses a screening method to prevent the precancerous lesions from developing into cervical cancer through early detection and treatment. Screening takes place through PAP smears, with three free PAP smears being offered to women reporting to the 12-hour unit. In the event of abnormal PAP smear results, patients are referred to the 24-hour unit for colposcopy. Colposcopy is the direct magnified inspection of the surface of a woman's cervix, using a light source and a microscope, to evaluate potentially cancerous areas, typically after an abnormal PAP smear. In some cases it may be best to treat the problem straightaway. This usually involves removing part of the cervix with a laser through a procedure called Large Loop Excision of the Transformational Zone (LLETZ). Research has revealed that HIV+ women have a 13% higher risk for developing cervical cancer than HIV–

women. Cervical cancer is now regarded as an AIDS-defining illness. At NCG, early management of cervical cancer is being reintroduced as a community service.

IT Infrastructure

Due to the poor telecommunication infrastructure that exists in the rural areas, localized support and infrastructure are essential for the smooth running of day-to-day operations. NCG relies on a computerised infrastructure to integrate its services and increase productivity. It includes biometric identification, barcode screening of pathology samples, internet, real-time web-based clinical software, and intranet. Connectivity for data communications between the sites and service providers is obtained through privately owned wireless networks. The local sites have large numbers of users who need to be supported on site.

Pharmacy

Institutional pharmacies fill prescriptions for all patients reporting to the ATC. These pharmacies are accredited with the SA Pharmacy Council and conform to Good Pharmacy Practice (GPP) guidelines.

Training Facility

NCG does extensive in-house, in-service, and external training and skills development. NCG's external training partners include the Foundation for Professional Development and Right-to-Care (both institutions offer PEPFAR-sponsored training courses), and NCG works closely with the universities of Utrecht, Pretoria, and UNISA through the Ndlovu Research Consortium. A full-time training & development manager supports line managers to identify skills and training gaps, and suggests how to bridge these gaps.

M&E Department with a Data-Capturing Unit

The M&E Department assists line managers to develop logical frameworks for reporting for all programmes. These logical frameworks identify inputs, outputs, outcomes, and activities that need to be attained in order to achieve the set objectives of the programmes. Please see the chapter on M&E (Chapter 4).

RAP Administration and Management

Each local site has decentralised services: IT, finance, M&E, and community liaison that assist operations. The central management team supplies the sites with specialised support services and ensures that sites are aligned and standardised (see Chapter 2 on Community Franchise Model).

5. Conclusion

The NCG ATC is a 'one-stop shop' for service delivery in rural areas. NCG's task is to integrate and support the District Health Care systems in cooperation with the Department of Health. Through PPPs, NCG is able to scale up these services in places without access to care. It is a service of excellence that remigrates skilled labour back to the rural areas and contributes to reducing the burden of disease by supplying the service where the treatment gap is biggest.

Through research and published articles, the NCG ATC concept has proven to have a long-term impact in its areas of function. It is with this track record in mind that we should like to see this model rolled out in more parts of the country as a solution to strengthen District Health Services delivery and to assist the Department of Health in its task at the national, provincial and district levels.

Notes

1. http://www.primaryhealthcare.uct.ac.za/approach/whatis/whatis.htm
2. http://www.hst.org.za/uploads/files/pocketguide.pdf
3. The Pocket Guide to District Health in South Africa, Health Systems Trust, 1997. http://www.healthlink.org.za/hst/isds
4. www.info.gov.za/speeches/2009/09060310551001.htm

References

Cohen, L., Chávez, V., & Chehimi, S. (2007). *Prevention is primary: Strategies for community well-being.* New York: Wiley.

Harrison, D. (1997). *Pocket Guide To District Health Systems in South Africa.* In: SA Health Review 2000. Paolo Alto, California: Healthwrights.

Morgan, W. P., & Goldston, S. E. (1987). *Exercise and mental health. The series in health psychology and behavioral medicine.* Washington, DC: Hemisphere Publishing Corp.

Spasoff, R.A., Harris, S.S., & Thuriaux, M.C. (2001). *A Dictionary Of Epidemiology.* Oxford: Oxford University Press.

US Preventive Services Task Force (Corporate Author) (1996). *Guide to Clinical Preventive Services: Report of the US Preventive Services Task Force.* Philadelphia: Lippincot, Williams & Wilkins.

WHO-UNICEF (1978). *Declaration of Alma-Ata.* International Conference on Primary Health USSR, 6-12 September. 1978. The International Conference on Primary Health Care (PHC).

Chapter 8

The 24-Hour Clinic: Maternal Care, Prevention of Mother-to-Child Transmission of HIV Infection (PMTCT), HIV & AIDS Inpatient Care

Robert Moraba[a]*, Hugo Tempelman*[b,c]*, Mariette Slabbert*[d]

"Labour is already a stressful environment. You are pregnant, poor, vulnerable, marginalized, uneducated. At that point, what do you rely on? What your mother told you when you left home? Your cultural beliefs, or this stranger who's standing there saying, 'Take this pill?'" 1

Abstract

As part of the Autonomous Treatment Centre (ATC), Ndlovu Care Group established a community-based, 24-hour clinic to complement the primary care services offered at the 12-hour clinic. The 24-hour clinic has three major components: (1) reproductive health, maternal and neonatal care, including community-based family planning, antenatal care, obstetrics, and postnatal follow-up programmes; (2) prevention of mother-to-child transmission (PMTCT) programme for HIV+ pregnant women; (3) TB/HIV & AIDS inpatient care that supports patients from the TB and HAART programmes who cannot be managed on an outpatient basis. Intermediate medical care and extensive nursing care with an emphasis on the nutritional status of these patients are pivotal. Through the ATC 24-hour clinic, NCG achieves its aims of tertiary prevention through the reduction of maternal death rates, reduction in neonatal mortality rate, prevention of mother to child transmission, and the rehabilitation of compromised HIV & AIDS patients.

1. Introduction

Maternal health refers to the health of women during pregnancy, childbirth and the postpartum period. While motherhood can be a positive and fulfilling experience, for too many women it is still associated with suffering, ill-health and even death, especially in developing countries. It is against this background that the 24-hour Mater-

---

a. Medical Director, Ndlovu 24-hour Clinic, Elandsdoorn, South Africa
b. CEO Ndlovu Care Group, Groblersdal, South Africa
c. Visiting Professor, Faculty of Social and Behavioural Sciences, Faculty of Medicine, Utrecht University, The Netherlands
d. COO Ndlovu Care Group, Groblersdal, South Africa

nity Clinic was built to service the community in the Moutse area, which is in dire need of essential services (Vermeer & Tempelman, 2008).

Most children living with HIV acquire the infection through mother-to-child transmission (MTCT), which can occur during pregnancy, labour, delivery and/or breastfeeding. Without specific interventions, HIV-infected women will pass the virus onto their infants during pregnancy or delivery in about 15-25% of cases; and an additional 5-20% of infants may become infected postnatally during breastfeeding, for an overall risk of 30-45% (WHO, UNAIDS, UNICEF & UNFPA, 2007).[2]

The risk of MTCT can be reduced to fewer than 2% by interventions that include (Dao et al., 2006):

– initiating antiretroviral (ARV) prophylaxis in the form of HAART, to reduce the viral load during labour to undetectable levels, continuing ART for one year after delivery, promoting exclusive breastfeeding as the preferred form of feeding[3];
– treating the infant during the first weeks of life, with a post-exposure prophylaxis (PEP) protocol;
– obstetrical interventions including elective caesarean delivery (prior to the onset of labour and rupture of membranes); and
– avoidance of mixed feeding (either exclusive breastfeeding or exclusive formula feeding) (Kagaavi, Gray, Brahmbhatt, et al., 2008).

The ultimate mission of the Ndlovu Care Group (NCG) maternal care and PMTCT programme is to eradicate paediatric HIV by preventing the transmission of HIV, at all entry points, using holistic maternal care. According to figures to date, the NCG PMTCT programme has managed to keep the transmission of HIV to newborns below 1%.[4]

When the HAART programme (free antiretroviral treatment roll-out programme) started in 2003, the first in Mpumalanga Province, a medical ward was added to the facility to provide comprehensive care, management, and treatment to patients who had advanced AIDS and/or severe complications. These services form part of the support for the patients in the HAART programme to make the care given holistic, integrated and community-based. Some 70% of patients with severe adverse events and opportunistic infections, and low CD4 counts, regain a quality of life with the inpatient care provided at the unit. The ATC 24-hour clinic has eight beds for the maternity department, with two delivery beds and a neonatal resuscitation unit. The medical ward also has eight beds, a four-bedded ward for men and one for women. In line with private hospital accreditation guidelines, the clinic is outfitted with sanitary and closet facilities, space for medical supplies and equipment storage, clean linen room, dietetic services and rehabilitation services. The unit is accredited with the National Department of Health as a private hospital and conforms to the R158 regulations.

The maternity clinic and medical section has a combined staff complement consisting of two midwives, one professional nurse, four enrolled nurses, four auxiliary nurses and four home-based health care workers. The home-based health care workers were trained in the facility after completing their theoretical studies. The staff is allocated to the medical section and the maternity section according to daily occupancy and patient care demands (acuity).

The aim of this chapter is to explain and elaborate on the activities and services that the 24-hour clinic provides, including maternal care, PMTCT and inpatient care for HIV & AIDS patients.

2. Maternal Care at the 24-Hour Unit

When the 24-hour unit was built in 1998, the aim was to achieve the goals, requirements, and quality standards set by the WHO. About 20-30 patients visit the clinic each day for antenatal and postnatal care. Pregnant women attending the unit come from various areas in Moutse East and the greater part of the former Kwa-Ndebele region. Each year, approximately 350 deliveries are done at the 24-hour unit, while about 8% of women, those presenting with obstructed labour, are referred to the nearest hospital with the request for a caesarean section[4]. The clinic is run by midwives who are supported by experienced medical practitioners. Labour records are well maintained and based on the labour graph in order to make timely decisions in case of delayed progress during labour. In the ten years that NCG ATC has provided this service to the community, the unit has had seven neonatal deaths and two maternal losses (HELLP syndrome and one amniotic fluid embolism).

The pregnancy and maternal care services provided at the unit follow the RAP continuum of care that includes prevention and retention programmes as described in Chapter 1. Services at the 24-hour unit include:

Primary prevention:
– Family planning;
– Routine antenatal care (ANC);
– Antenatal screening and care including VCT+;
– Maternity booking and planning of care;
– Obstetrical services.

Secondary prevention:
– Care for pre-existing medical conditions in pregnancy;
– Postnatal assessment and care for the neonate and the mother;
– Neonatal care and assessment;
– Infant feeding support and guidance;
– Promotion of healthy parent–infant relationships;
– Infection prevention and control in maternal care.

Tertiary prevention:
– Treating complications.

Retention:
– Adherence programmes for mothers initiated on treatment;
– Follow-up of babies to maintain HI-status.

The initiative serves as a model for new NCG ATCs in other rural areas in the country.

The 24-hour unit contributes to achieve Millennium Development Goals 4 and 5 (see Chapter 1) which are:

- Reduce child mortality
- Improve maternal health

These two goals seek to achieve the following targets:

Target 4a: Reduce by two-thirds the mortality rate among children under five
  4.1. Under-five mortality rate;
  4.2. Infant mortality rate;
  4.3. Proportion of 1-year-old children immunized against measles.

Target 5a: Reduce by three-quarters the maternal mortality ratio
  5.1. Maternal mortality ratio;
  5.2. Proportion of births attended by skilled health personnel.

Target 5b: Achieve, by 2015, universal access to reproductive health
  5.3. Contraceptive prevalence rate;
  5.4. Adolescent birth rate;
  5.5. Antenatal care coverage (at least one visit and at least four visits);
  5.6. Unmet need for family planning.

2.1. Primary Prevention

Family Planning

NCG offers family planning to guarantee:
- proper child spacing;
- prevent unwanted teenage and adult pregnancies;
- accurate information during counselling;
- awareness about sexually transmitted infections (STIs) for all patients presenting to the 12- and 24-hour clinics.

According to Family Health International, health policy-makers started to recognize the missed opportunities and lost efficiencies in the parallel approach of family planning services and VCT services. Family planning plays an important role in HIV & AIDS prevention and transmission, while VCT reaches clients who do not typically seek out family planning services as well as HIV+ women who wish to prevent unintended pregnancy. Integration of services also concentrates on family planning for increasing numbers of women of reproductive age, and a substantial unmet need for contraception.

Combining family planning and VCT services has the following benefits (FHI, 2008):
- Contraception is a key strategy in preventing MTCT of HIV, while VCT creates an opportunity to reach HIV+ women who wish to prevent unintended pregnancy.

- VCT attracts men and youth, who are not traditionally reached by family planning services.
- Delivery of family planning messages and services to VCT clients helps improve the utilisation and knowledge of contraceptives by reaching more people.
- There are cost efficiencies in combining services, assuming that clients need both services.

VCT provides an opportunity for a person to learn about and accept his or her HIV status in a confidential environment, where they can benefit from appropriate medical care and ongoing emotional support (UNAIDS, 2001). "Knowing your status" opens many avenues for women of childbearing age should they become HIV+. These avenues include PMTCT services, access to family planning, early medical care, access to peer & community support, availability of maternity services and planning for future need, such as care of orphans, dependents and the family. It has been shown that VCT results in more people returning for their test results and for repeat testing and counselling (Phanuphak, 2000).

The American College of Obstetrics and Gynaecology advocates that all women of childbearing age should receive preconception counselling as part of their routine primary care. This preconception counselling is aimed at providing education and counselling targeted at individual needs and identifying risk factors that may adversely affect maternal and fetal outcome. One of the very important risk factors is HIV infection. Unintended pregnancies occur at least 40% of the time, thus preconception counselling and testing for HIV will directly affect MTCT of HIV. An HIV-infected woman who has been identified should receive the following preconception counselling: selection of appropriate contraceptive methods, education about the perinatal transmission risks and ways to reduce the risks, evaluation and initiation of prophylaxis for opportunistic infections, optimization of maternal nutritional status, screening for STI, and initiation or modification of antiretrovirals (ARV), if available (Thisyakorn, Khongphatthanayothin, Sivichayakul, et al., 2000).

The importance of preconception counselling and testing is further illustrated in a report from Cote d'Ivoire about women who received VCT during pregnancy and who were subsequently diagnosed with HIV. In this study, the majority of women did not receive HIV results or care before delivery (Noba, Sibide, Kaba & Malkin, 2001).

For women who are already pregnant, VCT can help to provide an opportunity to discuss the different strategies to minimize the risk of perinatal transmission of HIV and to receive ongoing emotional support and medical care.

Routine Antenatal Care

NCG encourages women to come to the 24-hour unit as early in the pregnancy as possible. They will be enrolled in our ANC Clinic (antenatal care) and screened on intake for syphilis, anaemia, RH factor, blood glucose, routine urine test and VCT for HIV. During the intake visit, a routine ultrasound investigation will be performed to confirm the estimated gestational age of the fetus; this will be followed up during pregnancy in order to monitor fetal growth and congenital abnormalities.

Primigravida will be given, tetanus toxoid every semester and multipara, a booster once during the first antenatal visit. Tetanus toxoid is given to prevent tetanus from developing as a result of infection around the umbilical cord stump.

Follow-up visits are performed every four weeks to 32 weeks of pregnancy, then every two weeks to 36 weeks, and thereafter weekly consultations until delivery.

Clients receive multivitamins, ferrous sulphate and folic acid supplementation routinely at each visit.

During the antenatal care visits, a proper planning around the delivery will be facilitated with the assistance and input of the family members of the pregnant woman. A booking at our obstetric unit will be planned, and good after-care at home is discussed with the family members.

Obstetrical Services

Obstetric care begins with providing early, quality antepartum care. The moment a woman is in labour, she is expected to have transport arranged and to report immediately to the obstetric unit, she will be admitted, properly assessed, comforted and counselled for what is lying ahead. The aim is to deliver the baby vaginally, in a responsible way, for both HIV-negative and -positive women. Routine caesarean section for HIV+ pregnant women does not have a place in our protocols due to the initiation of HAART for viral suppression early in pregnancy. The obstetrical unit is run by a midwife supported by a doctor experienced in obstetrical care. The progress of labour is monitored using the labour graph. Risk-lines assist the midwife to make the proper decisions and call the doctor for his opinion if and when she sees fit. It is the doctor who finally decides to continue labour at the clinic or transfer the mother to the hospital for further obstetrical management.

For pregnant women who are HIV+, rupture of membranes more than 4 hours previously and invasive obstetric procedures such as amniocentesis and infant monitoring have been associated with an increased risk of transmission. A meta-analysis study showed that scheduled caesarean section (performed before the onset of labour and rupture of membranes) resulted in a 55-80% reduction in perinatal HIV transmission rates compared with emergency caesarean section and vaginal delivery regardless of ZDV use (The International Perinatal Group, 1999). However, the value of scheduled caesarean section in preventing perinatal HIV transmission in women who have low or undetectable viral load is unknown. The NCG 24-hour unit is not equipped to perform caesarean sections. Instead, mothers attending the antenatal care clinic at the 24-hour unit are initiated on HAART at 20 weeks' gestational age to suppress viral load during labour, in order to prevent transmission. Caesarean section is also associated with higher rates of complication including endometritis, wound infection, and pneumonia (The Perinatal HIV Guidelines Working Group, 2001).

2.2. Secondary Prevention

Care for pre-existing medical conditions in pregnancy

The most prevalent and most threatening pre-existing medical conditions during pregnancy are hypertension, diabetes mellitus, anaemia and STIs including HIV/AIDS. As described above, patients at the 24-hour unit are screened for all of these conditions during the first antenatal care visit. Proper protocols and management for each condition ensure that the underlying conditions will not have a negative impact on fetal development and growth or cause any obstetrical complication.

Prevention of Mother-to-Child Transmission

See under 4: the PMTCT services.

Postnatal Assessment and Care of the Neonate and Mother

After delivery, there is an intensive 24-hour observation phase:
– The mother's vital signs (blood pressure, temperature, etc.) are monitored, and possible obstetrical complications such as urine retention and postnatal haemorrhage are checked.
– Guidance is provided on how to properly breastfeed or, if formula feed is chosen, the correct preparation and administration of formula feed. The mother is instructed in the care of the umbilical cord and how to avoid infections. Proper hygiene instructions are given, including how these moments of care can be utilised for mother to neonate bonding. The neonate is fully examined after birth, BCG drops are given, chloramphenicol eye ointment is instilled, and urine and stool passage is checked.
– If the mother breastfeeds, she is given 200,000 units of Vitamin A upon discharge and 50,000 for non-breastfeeding neonates at six weeks postpartum. The PMTCT women stay longer in the unit so they can be educated in the preparation of the PEP with ARV-syrups for the neonate. A Road to Health card is filled in upon discharge and given to the mother.
– If everything is normal, the mother is discharged within 24 hours postpartum.

The mothers who attended our antenatal care are also offered postnatal care service (PNC). This is a comprehensive service lasting six weeks postpartum. Visits are made at three days, one week and six weeks after discharge.

Routine check-ups on neonatal jaundice, hygiene of the umbilical cord stump, breastfeeding, a well-contracted uterus, counselling around family planning, etc. belong to the PNC services.

2.3. Tertiary Prevention

Treating Complications

Because of the proper and standardized antenatal care clinic protocols, monitoring, and control of the pregnancy, complications are usually detected early. Even outside the normal ANC appointment dates, there is free access for those who have doubts or questions. Common complications such as urinary tract infections, hypertension, pregnancy-induced diabetes, etc. are usually diagnosed and treated before complications set in. Good protocols are in place to deal with pre-eclampsia or eclampsia, and an efficient referral system to the district government hospital ensures that patients with complications are treated at the appropriate level of care.

After birth, the most common complications are postpartum haemorrhage, urine retention, neonatal feeding problems and PEP administration problems.

2.4. Retention through Motivation

Adherence Programmes for Mothers Initiated on Treatment

Mothers that are initiated on ART are referred into the HAART programme where they join support groups and receive counselling at all visits. Please refer to Chapter 7.

Follow-up of Babies to Maintain HIV– Status

See below: The PMTCT services

3. The PMTCT Services: The NCG Approach

3.1. Objectives

The PMTCT services at NCG have as their objective the eradication of paediatric HIV through:
- Upon enrolment in the ANC programme, screening of all pregnant women for HIV and TB and offering a PAP smear to all pregnant HIV+ females.
- Ensuring the mother reaches undetectable viral load by time of birth by providing HAART.
- Reducing the risk of infection of the neonate (through the mother's blood and vaginal fluid during labour) by providing dual therapy as a post-exposure prophylaxis (PEP).

The NCG 24-hour clinic is an important entry point for *voluntary counselling and testing (VCT)* for pregnant women who report to the clinic for maternal care. This then leads to enrolment in the PMTCT programme and subsequent follow-up to the *highly active antiretroviral therapy (HAART)* after delivery of the baby. Through this link to child and maternal care, the mother is offered a lifelong continuum of care.

The PMTCT programme of NCG started in September 2003 and did not face many challenges as it was supported by a smoothly running maternity clinic and the HAART programme from the outset. The PMTCT programme was set against the global inequities of HIV: More than 95% of paediatric HIV infections occur in resource-limited settings, while HIV transmission rates in infants in developed countries where PMTCT is practised is reported to be The low coverage and uptake in resource-limited settings show that (Chaturvedi & Chaturvedi, 2008):
— Less than 15% of pregnant women are tested for HIV;
— Less than 10% are offered ARV prophylaxis;
— Less than 5% of HIV+ women in need of treatment are offered ART.

NCG's primary prevention strategy in the PMTCT programme entails:
— prevention of HIV in prospective parents;
— offering VCT+ to all pregnant women;
— prevention of unintended pregnancies among HIV+ women.

Secondary and tertiary prevention is achieved through HIV & AIDS, TB, chronic disease, and STI screening for all pregnant women to detect infection and co-morbidities early.

3.2. *Principles*

At the NCG 24-hour clinic, HAART is started at a gestational age of 20 weeks, regardless of the maternal CD4 count, to ensure viral suppression by the time labour occurs, with the following regimen: AZT/3TC/NVP, and normal vaginal delivery is done if possible. To control the NVP toxicity, there is special emphasis on the liver enzymes during the pregnancy period. The antenatal care clinic schedule for both HIV+ and HIV– pregnant women is exactly the same. The follow-up period for neonate and mother postpartum is one year due to the one-year PCR confirmation of the infant's HIV status.

3.3. *Postpartum Care*

Postpartum care includes:
— HIV+ mothers stay 3-4 days in the unit for training on how to give PEP medication to the neonate.
— The neonate starts PEP dual therapy (AZT/3TC).
— The mother is advised to breastfeed exclusively.
— Maternal ART is continued for preferably 1 year.
— If the baseline CD4 at the start of the mother's antenatal care is below 350 cells/ml, ARVs are continued lifelong, and if baseline CD4 is above 350 cells/ml, NVP is stopped after a year, tailing off the AZT/3TC over a period of four more days.
— The mother remains in the programme with bi-annual CD4 count checkups and counselling. When she is eligible for ARVs, she will be enrolled for lifelong management in the HAART retention programme.

3.4. Neonate

The neonate is given PEP: AZT/3TC for one month. The laboratory monitoring of the baby includes two full blood counts for the detection of AZT-induced anaemia, together with a PCR at week six, to be confirmed after one year. The one-year follow-up is difficult to execute due to non-compliance of the mother/caregiver.

3.5. Women Who Did Not Attend Antenatal Clinic at the 24-hour Maternity Clinic

A VCT is done upon admission before delivery and, if the test is positive, followed by once-off NVP during delivery, after which HAART is initiated if indicated. Immediately postpartum, full HIV staging of the mother is done. The protocol for the neonate remains the same.

4. HIV & AIDS Inpatient Care

The term 'hospice' (from the same linguistic root as 'hospitality') can be traced back to medieval times when it referred to a place of shelter and rest for weary or ill travellers on a long journey.[5] The name was first applied to specialized care for dying patients in 1967 by the physician Dame Cicely Saunders, who founded the first modern hospice, St. Christopher's Hospice, in a residential suburb of London.

In contrast to typical hospices, the NCG ATC 24-hour unit focuses not only on caring, but also on curing and management of:
- opportunistic infections,
- complications at the start of ART, and
- the patient in the cachectic phase.

These patients are dependent on their surroundings for survival, and in most cases, patients who are admitted as terminal to the unit are discharged to lead a normal life.

In NCG's experience, patients who are referred to hospitals with full-blown AIDS, severe tuberculosis or both are often refused hospital access and are sent home for terminal care. The treatment provided in this unit often makes the difference between life and death, with a good outcome for approximately 62% of the patients admitted. The mortality of these patients is high, namely 38%,[4] as they are severely compromised upon admission. After discharge from the 24-hour clinic, patients are referred to the NCG HAART programme through which the continuum of lifelong care is guaranteed.

Considered the model for quality, compassionate care for people facing a life-limiting/threatening illness or injury, hospice and palliative care involve a team-oriented approach to expert medical care, pain management, and emotional and spiritual support expressly tailored to the patient's needs and wishes. Support is provided to the patient's loved ones as well.

Palliative care extends the principles of hospice care to a broader population that could benefit from receiving this type of care earlier in their illness or disease process. No specific therapy is excluded from consideration, but care excludes life support and resuscitation. An individual's needs are continually assessed, and treatment options are explored and evaluated in the context of the individual's values and symptoms.

How Does Hospice & Palliative Care Work?

Typically, a family member serves as the primary caregiver and, when appropriate, helps make decisions with the ill individual. Staff members nurse and care for the patient and provide additional care and other services. The unit functions 24 hours a day, seven days a week. The team develops a care plan that meets each patient's individual needs for pain management and symptom control. The team usually consists of a doctor, nurses, care workers and counsellors.

What Services Are Provided?

Among its major responsibilities, the interdisciplinary team:
— manages the patient's illness, pain and symptoms;
— assists the patient with physical, emotional and psychosocial support;
— provides needed drugs, medical supplies, and equipment;
— coaches the family on how to care for the patient;
— delivers special services like rehabilitation and physical therapy when needed;
— arranges short- to medium-term inpatient care as necessary.

4.1. Pain Management

For inpatients who are bedridden, pain control is very important. Patients and caregivers are trained in pain control. The medication used is often limited to what is affordable; combinations of paracetamol, NSAIDs and codeine often provide the required relief. If needed, opiates are administered in the form of syrups and tablets.

4.2. Food and Nutrition

The nutritional needs of the patient change due to morbidity depending on the opportunistic illness. The health care team helps the patient and family to understand why certain foods are given or omitted. In our inpatient facility, the full-blown AIDS patients are often too weak to feed themselves. At that point, the family contribution in assisting the patient with feeding is invaluable. Spoon for spoon, sip by sip is a time-consuming process for busy clinical staff, and patients often do not get what they deserve in the hospital setting. This is another reason why NCG advocates decentralization of these services in order to create easy access for the family to assist without incurring logistics problems and additional cost.

4.3. Support for the Patient

This holistic approach ensures that the patient and the family receive attention concerning all aspects of the medical treatment, expected outcome and continued care after discharge, and that the family understands and adheres to the treatment protocol. The treatment protocol includes the risk assessment and the support required from the family for the initial treatment period. Family members are also counselled.

4.4. Hydration of the Patient

Patients who are severely ill need proper hydration with monitoring of input and output of fluids. Proper fluid therapy management is essential. The medical care needed for these patients is often beyond the capabilities of the general practitioners working in the centre. The 24-hour unit is supported with the knowledge and experience of a senior specialist in infectious diseases who advises and educates staff in the advanced management of the complicated problems they are faced with.

5. Cervical Cancer Programme

Since 1997, over 33,000 women have died of cervical cancer in South Africa. This translates into roughly 3,000 per year. In addition, approximately 7,000 women develop the disease every year.[6] In 2000, a national cervical cancer screening policy was developed and put into place. The policy advocates screening with a PAP smear to detect the precancerous lesions. Referral and follow-up prevent the precancerous lesions from developing into cervical cancer. Three free PAP smears are offered to women in public service at the ages of 30, 40 and 50. This policy was then viewed as the most rational approach to ensure the widest coverage for all women in South Africa.[6]

Statistics suggest that since its implementation, less than 20% of women have accessed this service. At present, there are approximately 5.7 million people living with HIV & AIDS in South Africa, of which 60% are women.[6] Researchers have identified an increase in morbidity and mortality due to cancer of the cervix associated with HIV & AIDS. Research has revealed that HIV+ women have a 13% greater risk of developing cervical cancer than HIV– women. This risk increases as the immunological status of the patient deteriorates. Cervical cancer is now regarded as an AIDS-defining illness.[6]

As the national cervical cancer screening policy was established before the link between cervical cancer and HIV & AIDS was firmly established, there is currently a gap in the cervical screening policy. While the need for cervical cancer services is addressed in the HIV & AIDS/STI National Strategic Plan 2007-2011, it is not clearly articulated or completely integrated within the broad range of services that would constitute an effective response to these twin diseases. It is suggested that as women are living longer due to access to HAART, they are at an increased risk of contracting cervical cancer. Both cervical cancer and HIV are sexually transmitted diseases with no immediate visible symptoms. Cervical cancer originates from a sexually transmitted agent called human papillomavirus (HPV), which silently grows in the cervix and later becomes invasive. The difference between cervical cancer in HIV & AIDS-positive and HIV-negative women is that HIV+ women commonly contract invasive cancer ten years earlier than women who are HIV–.[6]

At the NCG there is a treatment protocol for screening, diagnosis, staging, and management of early-stage cervical cancer. The enabling diagnostics for including cervical screening as part of the comprehensive care package is a colposcope and a LETTZ laser. Our medical professionals have been trained in this service by experienced gynaecological oncologists. In this way, early management of cervical cancer is reintroduced as a community service.[6]

6. Conclusion

The success of the 24-hour clinic hinges on all the major components of the integrated NCG model, with concerted efforts from logistics and decision-making. The 12-hour clinic as point of entry delivers integrated PHC, tuberculosis, HIV & AIDS care, which people can visit when they are in need of primary care. The compromised patients and women who are pregnant are referred to the 24-hour clinic for procedures such as VCT+ and routine antenatal care. The cervical screening and treatment programme restores early oncology management to a community level in a responsible manner. This has become a medical priority given that HPV infection is a co-infection of HIV, resulting in the development of cervical cancer as an AIDS-defining illness.

The 24-hour unit is an asset in the community, bringing back essential services to local level, and it reduces the workload for the district hospital tremendously.

Notes

1. New York Times (6 August 2006), *"When a Pill Is Not Enough"*.
2. http://www.who.int
3. WHO PMTCT Guidelines 2009
4. Data retrieved from existing local NCG databases
5. http://www.nhpco.org/i4a/pages/index.cfm?pageid=3285
6. http://www.righttocare.org

References

Chaturvedi, S.K., & Kanupriya Chaturvedi (2008). *Antiretroviral Drugs for Treating Pregnant Women and Preventing HIV Infection in Infants in Resource-Limited Settings.* Geneva: WHO.

Dao, H., Mofenson, L.M., Ekpini, R., Gilks, C.F., Barnhart, M., Bolu, O., & Shaffer, N. (2006). *International recommendations on antiretroviral drugs for treatment of HIV-infected women and prevention of mother-to-child HIV transmission in resource-limited settings. Update.* Atlanta, GA (USA): Centers for Disease Control and Prevention; National Center for HIV, Hepatitis, STD, TB Prevention.

FHI (2008). *Report: Integrating Family Planning into HIV Voluntary Counselling and Testing Services in Kenya: Progress to Date and Lessons Learned.* Found at http://fhi.org.

The International Perinatal Group (1999). The mode of delivery and the risk of vertical transmission of human immunodeficiency virus type 1 - a metaanalysis of 15 prospective cohort studies. *New England Journal of Medicine, 340*, 977-987.

Kagaayi, J., Gray, R.H., Brahmbhatt, H., Kigozi, G., Nalugoda, F., Wabwire-Mangen, F., Serwadda, D., Sewankambo, N., Ddungu, V., Ssebagala, D., Sekasanvu, J., Makumbi, F., Kiwanuka, N., Lutalo, T., Reynolds, S.J., & Wawer, M.J. (2008). *Survival of Infants Born to HIV-Positive Mothers by Feeding Modality, in Rakai, Uganda.* PLoS One. 2008; 3(12):e3877. Epub 2008 Dec 9. PMCID: PMC2588542.

Noba, V., Sidibe, K., Kaba, F., & Malkin, J.E (2001). Voluntary screening and prevention of mother-to-child transmission of HIV among pregnant women in Cote d'Ivoire: A public health program of the international therapeutic solidarity fund (ITSF). *Proceedings of the 8th Conference on Retroviruses and Opportunistic Infections (Abstract 704)*. Chicago, February 4-8, 2001.

The Perinatal HIV Guidelines Working Group (2001). *Public health service task force recommendations for use of antiretroviral drugs in pregnant HIV-1 infected women for maternal health and interventions to reduce perinatal HIV-1 transmission in the United States*. January 24, 2001. Published online: www.hivatis.org.

Phanuphak, P. (2000). Voluntary Counseling and Testing. *Proceedings of the UNAIDS Regional Task Force Meeting, Phnom Penh*. Cambodia, May 10-12, 2000.

Thisyakorn, U., Khongphatthanayothin, M., Sivichayakul, S., Rongkavilit, C., Poolcharoen, W., Kunanusont, C., Bien, D.D., & Phanuphak, P. (2000). Thai Red Cross zidovudine donation program to prevent vertical transmission of HIV: the effect of the modified ACTG 076 regimen. *AIDS, 14*, 2921-7.

UNAIDS (2001). *Document: Mother-to-Child Transmission of HIV - Technical Update, 2, 25*.

Vermeer, A., & Tempelman, H. (Eds.) (2008). *Health Care in Rural South Africa: an Innovative Approach (Third, revised and extended edition)*. Amsterdam: VU University Press.

WHO, UNAIDS, UNICEF & UNFPA (2007). *HIV Transmission Through Breastfeeding, A Review of Available Evidence: 2007 Update*. WHO Library Cataloguing-in-Publication Data.

Chapter 9

The 12-Hour Clinic: Integrated Primary Health, TB and HAART Care

Hugo Tempelman[a,b], *Mariette Slabbert*[c], *Peter Schrooders*[d], *Kedumetse Mvula*[e], *Phiwa Sondlane*[f]

Abstract

Chronic diseases are no longer viewed as distinct or isolated health problems and should not be treated as such. The latest approach to treating and preventing chronic conditions emphasizes the impact of the disease on the quality of life of the person and his/her family and evaluates the type of approach in terms of the effect on the health system. Consequently, the 12-hour clinic of the Ndlovu Care Group Autonomous Treatment Centre delivers holistic primary care in a decentralised rural setting as part of the Rural Advancement Plan. The 12-hour clinics operate autonomously inside the community, and its healthcare model is designed according to the primary, secondary and tertiary principles of prevention. In this chapter the focus is on the implementation of integrated primary health, TB and HAART care, the facilitations through IT and technology, and the opportunities that the lessons learned from the double epidemic provides to improve primary care service delivery.

1. Introduction

The World Health Organisation publication, *Innovative Care for Chronic Conditions* (2002),[1] states that from a healthcare perspective, it is no longer advantageous to view chronic conditions as discrete health problems, nor according to the traditional categories of non-communicable and communicable diseases. The report argues that innovative care is not based on the aetiology of a particular problem but on the demands that the health problem places on the healthcare system. In the case of chronic conditions, the demands are similar regardless of the cause of the condition. Moreover, effective management strategies are remarkably comparable for many

a. CEO Ndlovu Care Group, Groblersdal, South Africa
b. Visiting Professor, Faculty of Social and Behavioural Sciences, Faculty of Medicine, Utrecht University, The Netherlands
c. CEO Ndlovu Care Group, Groblersdal, South Africa
d. Medical Director Ndlovu Medical Centre, Elandsdoorn, South Africa
e. Manager HAART & TB Programme Ndlovu Care Group, Elandsdoorn, South Africa
f. Manager ARV Programme, Ndlovu Care Group, Elandsdoorn, South Africa

chronic problems, and inclusive chronic conditions management is developing an identity of its own in health care.

In new conceptualizations of chronic conditions, the quality of life of the patient and family is considered an important outcome, and the role of the patient in producing this outcome is emphasized. The patient is not an inactive participant in care and should take responsibility for his/her own well-being through active participation in the management of the condition he/she suffers from or its prevention.

The Alma Ata Declaration on Primary Health Care (WHO-UNICEF, 1978) defines primary health care (PHC) as "essential health care based on practical, scientifically sound and socially acceptable methods and technology, made universally accessible to individuals and families in the community through their full participation and at a cost that the community and the country can afford to maintain at every stage of their development in the spirit of self-reliance and self-determination".

According to the Faculty of Health Sciences, University of Cape Town,[2] PHC is therefore understood as an approach to health care that promotes the attainment by all people of a level of health that will permit them to live socially and economically productive lives. It is health care that is essential, scientifically sound (evidence-based), ethical, accessible, equitable, affordable, and accountable to the community. In other words, it is not only primary medical or curative care, nor is it a package of low-cost medical interventions for the poor and marginalised. On the contrary, it calls for the integration of health services in the process of community development, a process that requires political commitment, intersectoral collaboration, and multi-disciplinary involvement for success.

The Ndlovu Care Group (NCG) 12-hour clinics deliver holistic primary care in a decentralised rural setting, viewing comprehensive health as an essential element in advancing the rural communities they operate in.

The NCG's Autonomous Treatment Centres (ATCs) operate inside the community and base their health care model on the primary, secondary and tertiary principles of prevention, to provide sustainable and affordable community-based health. Patient commitment and compliance to long-term treatment plans are maximised through retention programmes that motivate individuals. In line with the definitions of primary, secondary, and tertiary prevention described in Chapter 1, the 12-hour units strive to deliver services that promote:

– *Primary prevention*: Informed clients will prevent themselves or their families falling ill in the first place. This means that the community as a whole needs to be informed about nutrition, lifestyle, substance abuse, etc. that can induce certain chronic diseases (hypertension, obesity, diabetes mellitus, cardiovascular diseases, etc.). It is therefore important that the community recognises the early signs and symptoms of illness, that the community is screened and tested for underlying/latent diseases, and that patients are staged in terms of disease progression and provided with a management plan. This approach also requires behavioural change to ensure long-term outcomes.

– *Secondary prevention*: accessible services that promote early care-seeking behaviour in individuals. This is necessary to ensure that mild symptoms and opportunistic infections are managed before they cause serious disease or adversity like job losses, disability or incapacity.

– *Tertiary prevention*: equipped and resourced facilities that can offer quality decentralised care to the population to minimise morbidity and mortality.
– *Retention through motivation*: intensive adherence counselling, monitoring and evaluation, feedback on progress, and access to other development and motivation programmes that reinforce compliance with treatment plans.

2. Tuberculosis in South Africa

For many years, South Africa's HIV & AIDS epidemic has been the focus of international attention. This has been discussed in depth in Chapter 3. Moreover, high rates of HIV infection elicited questions regarding the sexual culture, socio-economic conditions and biomedical realities of the so-called 'rainbow nation'.

While the attention focused on HIV was duly warranted, another epidemic has remained largely ignored. Nevertheless, it has an intimate connection with HIV morbidity and mortality, and important questions are posed by the interactions between the two diseases. HIV is a relatively new disease in South Africa, with the first deaths due to AIDS occurring in 1982. However, tuberculosis (TB) has a much longer history, reflecting the industrial and demographic processes which shaped South Africa's past and which continue to impact the health of the population at large.

The poor performance of TB control programmes and many years of low cure rates have seen the emergence of drug-resistant strains of the disease that are more difficult and costly to diagnose and treat; the caseload of drug-resistant TB now puts South Africa among the world's top 10 countries. In a recent outbreak of extensively drug-resistant TB (XDR-TB) in HIV-infected patients in South Africa, half of the infections were acquired in clinics and hospitals, and included healthcare workers (Benater, 2004). The mortality rate exceeded 95%[3]. National incidence rates are escalating, and in 2006, the World Health Organisation (WHO) estimated that there were 940 cases of TB for every 100,000 people in South Africa. The WHO recently ranked South Africa fourth among the world's 22 high-burden TB countries in terms of absolute case numbers[4]. The African continent, which accounts for only 11% of the world's population[5], is currently responsible for 29% of the global burden of TB cases and 34% of related deaths. More than half a million people in Africa die each year of TB.

With its history of inequitable distribution of resources and health facilities, South Africa has long shouldered a heavy disease burden of TB. The migrant labour system, in which miners lived and worked in cramped, unsanitary conditions in between visits to their home communities across South Africa, provided fertile conditions for the emergence and entrenchment of a national TB epidemic[6]. The interaction of TB and HIV in South Africa requires far greater attention and research. Put broadly, however, the rapid spread of HIV across South Africa during the early 1990s is partly attributable to the high national prevalence of TB and its weakening impact on the general immunity of the population. The confluence of these diseases also works in opposite directions, with the biomedical effects of HIV resulting in higher TB caseloads and more virulent TB infections. Approximately 53% of South Africans with TB are also HIV-positive[7], with dual infection rates of up to 80% in some communities

(Gandhi, Moll, Pawinski et al., 2006). HIV infection increases the risk of developing TB tenfold.

HIV treatment efforts could be boosted through routine testing at all healthcare facilities and raising the threshold for starting antiretroviral treatment to a CD4 cell count of 350. This was implemented in South Africa in March 2010. This political decision is the best TB prevention intervention this country has implemented in the last 25 years. HIV treatment programmes play an important part in prevention: studies show that patients who start antiretroviral treatment early are less likely to transmit the virus, less likely to contract TB and more likely to access sexual and reproductive health services.

Failure to diagnose and treat TB promptly leads to ongoing transmission of the airborne infection and increased deaths, particularly in those whose immune systems have been weakened by HIV infection. The most commonly used test in Africa – the sputum smear – does not work well to detect TB in HIV-infected patients. Even with the right diagnosis and successful treatment of TB, the cure rate for the disease is 70%, far below the World Health Organisation goal of 85%.

With the political turn South Africa took in 2008-2009, more attention is being focused on the TB epidemic in South Africa.[8] However, what is needed is a massive budget scale-up for TB services in conjunction with the establishment and implementation of what is known in public health as the 'Three 'I'[9]. These are:

(1) Intensified Case Finding

Intensified Case Finding involves TB contact screening and screening of all HIV-positive patients for TB at least every six months. The Department of Health reports that around 40% of HIV patients are screened for TB, while the World Health Organisation estimates this to be less than 1% for South Africa. Regardless of the alarming discrepancies in these statistics, what is certain is that screening must be dramatically increased if deaths from AIDS and TB co-infection are to be reduced.

At the NCG 12-hour clinics, medical personnel, counsellors and fieldworkers perform TB screenings on all patients that report to the clinic and at all levels in the community where there is or was client/provider contact.

The criteria used for TB contact screenings are:
– household contacts of patients diagnosed with smear-positive pulmonary TB;
– patients who live within the designated project target areas;
– all children under 5 years of age;
– all patients who report to the clinics;
– all individuals who undergo HIV counselling and testing.

All HIV-positive patients are also screened for TB before they start HAART and at every visit to the clinic. As soon as a patient is screened and identified as a TB suspect, or diagnosed with TB, they will immediately be evaluated and TB treatment started. Counselling and psychosocial assessment are performed to ensure that the patient is ready and committed to start six months of uninterrupted treatment. Patients receive TB treatment training before they start taking the medication to ensure that:

- the patient understands the commitment and is willing to take the treatment as prescribed;
- the patient will recognize and know how to manage or report the treatment side effects;
- the patient will appoint a *treatment assistant*, often a family member, who will help and support him/her at home.

During the course of the treatment, the patient will receive ongoing counselling, clinical monitoring, and treatment support during each clinic visit.

(2) Effective Infection Control Policy

Improving infection control is an imperative, as nosocomial TB transmission (in the healthcare setting) is common at South African healthcare sites. As the public antiretroviral treatment (ART) roll-out gains momentum, increasing attention is being paid to the interaction of HIV and TB, and of the effects of the ART roll-out on the latter. An article on TB infection control in resource-limited settings has outlined the ways in which the very treatment initiatives created by the scale-up of ART have created 'unprecedented opportunities' for immune-suppressed patients to be exposed to TB within healthcare facilities (Bock, Jensen, Miller & Nardell, 2007).

(3) Isoniazid Preventative Therapy (IPT)

A roll-out of IPT as a prophylactic measure could reduce the risk of HIV-positive people developing TB by more than 65%, thereby dramatically decreasing HIV/TB mortality. IPT has been prescribed to only 4% of HIV-positive people in South Africa. The state is therefore failing to provide this essential prophylaxis.

HIV-positive healthcare workers risk their own health when they treat patients with active TB, they reduce the productivity of the healthcare facility if they contract TB, and they could simultaneously present a TB infection risk to their other patients[9].

As the ART roll-out drives the establishment of new primary healthcare facilities in resource-limited countries, new healthcare sites are designed and built. Building plans and renovations must consider TB infection control as integral to the construction of new healthcare facilities to ensure optimal natural ventilation[10].

3. Holistic Primary Care Service Delivery

The 12-hour clinic in Elandsdoorn started as a private general medical practice in 1994, Ndlovu Medical Centre, in an area with no other clinical or essential services available. From patient records, it soon became evident that the same patients were returning to the clinic on a regular basis but presented with different ailments every time. This alerted the practice to the fact that the patients were also suffering from 'poverty' and its associated consequences like malnutrition, lack of education, and unemployment, apart from general ailments and complaints. It is from this premise that the community development projects were created to support the clinic to serve the community with integrated community health and community care programmes, or the Rural Advancement Plan as it is now referred to, to ensure a holistic approach.

According to the WHO Innovative Care for Chronic Conditions report, 2002[11], the poor are at risk of becoming more impoverished when they experience diminished health or a health crisis in the household. They often spiral in a vicious cycle of poverty and poor health. This cycle involves:
- limited resources to purchase food, sanitation, and healthcare, which leads to
- impoverished health, which in turn leads to
- reduced capacity to work and lowered productivity,
- this further decreases the resources to purchase food, sanitation, and healthcare, and so on.

The report claims that a cycle such as this one is difficult to break and often perpetuates. In families in which a parent has a chronic condition that precludes his/her working, children are at risk of poor health due to the lack of family resources, and when they surrender to illness, the cycle of poverty and chronic health problems endures. The children develop chronic disabling conditions, cannot participate in the work force as adults, cannot purchase resources, and are unable to improve their health or poverty situation. When they have children, the cycle continues.

The report also explores the path from poverty to chronic conditions; it recognises that a number of socio-environmental factors play a role and are critical determinants of health status:
- *Prenatal Factors* (Blackwell, Hayward & Crimmins, 2001; Law, Egger, Dada et al., 2001; Law, de Swiet, Osmond et al., 1993): Mothers with poor nutritional standing bear children who experience chronic conditions in adulthood such as diabetes, hypertension, and heart disease. Poverty and poor health during childhood are associated with adult chronic conditions as well, including cancer, pulmonary disease, cardiovascular disease, and arthritis.
- *Ageing* (Dranga, 1997; Lynch, Kaplan, Shema et al., 2001; Zimmer, 2001): The role of age surfaces in studies of the impoverished elderly in developed and developing countries.
- *Education and Unemployment* (Ali, Khalid, Pirkani, 1989; Ludermir & Lewis, 2001; Robins, Locke & Regier, 1991): Poor families tend to receive less education, which has been associated with higher rates of mental disorders in Brazil and linked in Pakistan with limited knowledge of chronic conditions and their management. Moreover, unemployment has been associated with health problems; morbidity and mortality rates are higher in the unemployed than in the general population.
- *Environment* (Cohen, 2000; Marmot & Bobak, 2001; Mengesha & Bekele, 1989; Narayan, Chambers, Shah et al., 2000; Tomatis, 2001;Warden, 1989): Environments where the poor live and work are associated with diminished health status. Greater exposure to disease agents, increased susceptibility, and poor health behaviours interact to impact their health status. The work environments of the poor tend to be more physically demanding and place individuals at risk of injury due to automobile collisions or exposure to harmful substances. Hazardous chemical

exposure and pollution, particularly in developing countries, have been linked to local prevalence rates of cancer, cardiovascular, and respiratory diseases.
– *Access to care* (Asch, Sloss, Hogan et al., 2000; Ensor & San, 1996; Chernichovsky & Meesook, 1986; Gao, Tang, Tolhurst et al., 2001; Leyva-Flores, Kageyama & Erviti-Erice, 2001; Nyonator & Kutzin, 1999; Stierle, Kaddar, Tchicaya et al., 1999): The economically impoverished often lack access to health care or preventive measures that, in turn, have been associated with poor health outcomes and exacerbation of chronic conditions. Care is often delayed or impeded because of the cost for indigent groups. In general, preventive care is too costly and often out of reach for the poor, allowing avoidable health problems to become chronic conditions. Finally, even when care is publicly funded, distance and travel time may exclude the poor from receiving adequate services.

The report then explores the path from chronic conditions to poverty and concludes that the poverty-chronic condition relationship is bi-directional; loss of income, the cost of treatment, and marginalisation because of chronic health problems negatively affect the economic status of those with chronic conditions.

NCG initiated a TB programme in a pioneering public-private partnership with the Mpumalanga Department of Health in 1997. In March 2005 the programme received full support from the South African National Department of Health, viz. the National Tuberculosis Control Programme,[12] that included TB data collection and recording tools (i.e. ETR, registers, patient cards, etc.), active M&E and visible support at the district and sub-district level. This innovative public-private partnership was an unique achievement in those days.

In 2003, the 12-hour clinic in Elandsdoorn expanded its services to start a Dutch-funded ART rollout programme at the clinic. PEPFAR funding replaced the Dutch sponsor in 2004, and in 2009 the HAART and TB programmes were accredited with the National Department of Health as comprehensive management care and treatment rollout sites. In the absence of funding, the primary healthcare part still operates as a private practice to provide integrated care to the community.

With the development of the partnerships described above, the problem arose of how to deliver the service in a comprehensive way. NCG therefore developed strategies based on a few sound questions: How do we prevent disease, how do we identify it early, how do we restore the faith of the public in disease management, how can technology enable the service delivery in rural areas, how do we keep chronic patients compliant with their treatment protocols? The first two questions will be extensively dealt with in Part Three of this book.

It is NCG's view that an adequate response to health-related problems at all levels will make the public aware that disease can be prevented, that disease can be interdicted even if it is already present, and that disease should not be stigmatised. It is also our belief that personalising the prevention, care, treatment, and compliance builds and restores faith in service delivery; that consistent messaging creates reliability and credibility; and that easy access to care removes the threshold to disclosing problems and attending the clinic. The community CHAMP programme (discussed in Part Three) is therefore an extremely important component of community mobilisation, destigmatisation, awareness and behavioural change.

At the 12-hour clinics we try to restore their confidence in good service delivery through the implementation of the comprehensive National Department of Health strategic plans. We destigmatise disease by integrating services and disease management; all patients are treated holistically rather than in separate programmes. We also destigmatise through creating awareness and mobilising the community to identify and convince individuals to come for screening for underlying disease and to report to the clinic. There are no special clinic days for mono-disease management but an integrated service delivery. This means that a client suffering from multiple medical problems is managed in one clinic visit and does not have to come on separate special days for his/her HIV problems, TB management and diabetes treatment. In the 12-hour clinic we personalise services by booking the client with his/her own preferred healthcare provider of choice. This implies that there is an effort made for PHC and/ or chronic disease clients to have the same healthcare provider on consecutive visits in order to build a relationship of trust. This also has the spin-off that the healthcare provider follows the client over time and has a better perspective in managing all his/ her co-morbidities. It also gives the healthcare provider pride in his/her professional efforts and acts as a motivator. The privacy of patients is respected, and all consultations including sputum collection are performed confidentially.

Strict infection control measures and policies are implemented, and all waiting areas are open, ventilated and outside. Waste disposal is integrated in these policies, with sharp incineration in each cubicle and medical waste incineration on the premises.

Technology was introduced at an early stage in NCG's model of care. It has to support and enable the user rather than frustrate him/her. This implies that training goes hand in hand with the introduction of technology for all levels of personnel. The introduction of technology should be motivated by the improvement it can make in a process. It started simply and developed from there:
- The introduction of a fax machine made it possible to fax an ECG to a cardiologist in order to import specialist knowledge to support the general practitioner in the field, improving the level of service to the patient.
- Digital photographs of certain skin lesions were emailed to a dermatologist, and the resulting interpretation brought specialist diagnosis back to the rural setting.
- Video recording of ultrasound findings created an environment in which our health professionals could improve their interpretation skills through distance learning.
- Digital X-rays can be emailed, and on-site teaching through specialist opinion per email improved the service.
- IT management systems for patient registration and stock management in the pharmacy were introduced.

This phased approach had its pros and cons. The fragmentation of IT-related issues can result in multiple, sometimes incompatible databases, difficult reconciliations and increased workload. The introduction of technology allows task shifting to

lower-level and therefore more affordable employees to save on programme cost without compromising quality. This opened the door for an integrated Electronic Health Management System:
- patient registration;
- identification and management;
- clinic flow and integrated services;
- ICD10 coding integrated in diagnoses;
- pharmacy protocols and billing;
- stock control;
- laboratory services and other diagnostics, connected to
- monitoring & evaluation for project management and reporting.

NCG was actively looking for a solution to provide the possibility of integrated service management for large numbers of patients in a well-controlled environment. As part of its social responsibility programme, Anglo American made an in-house-developed system called the Health Source available to NCG. This system provides IT management for PHC/TB/HIV treatment and care for the individual and specialised cohorts. It is web-based and gives the patient the possibility to migrate between clinics and its main service provider. It is the aim of both partners to develop this system as an example of how user-friendly electronic health management systems can support disease management, how they can improve programme evaluation, how they can serve as a tool to improve the local implementation of services, and how they can be of assistance to the government for use in the public sector.

The South African infrastructure on IT and digitalisation created a robust environment for the introduction of IT technology, even in the most rural areas. Data transfer through mobile phone technology, copper cable, fibre optics or satellite is all within reach.

Examples of NCG's improvement of services through the implementation of IT are:
- *Diagnostic Imaging Department:*
  The Digital X-ray Department has taken a few logistical problems out of the equation. No longer problems because of being out of stock of films, developer and/or fixative. No longer storage problems of X-rays and patient files. Expert specialist knowledge at hand through service emailing X-rays to the radiology departments we liaise with. Ultrasound imaging live-recordings is another example of how specialist knowledge can be obtained in the rural areas, improving the diagnostic possibilities through the implementation of technology.
- *HIV Monitoring Laboratory:*
  The existing NCGs have a HIV monitoring laboratory on site which are managed by medical technologists. They are qualified to perform the tests but not to sign off on the results. Data transfer in daily batches to the main laboratory where specialist pathologists are employed creates the possibility to sign off at a distance and have the approved and properly interpreted results returned to the rural facility.

— *Retention Programmes:*

As discussed before, it is the NCG's opinion that patients share the responsibility for their own well-being with us. It is not only the service provider who has that responsibility, and similarly, chronic disease management is a two-way responsibility. The provider has the responsibility to deliver consistent and appropriate quality care without stock-outs, treatment interruption, or lack of service delivery. The client has a responsibility regarding behavioural change, treatment compliance and prevention of disease progress through lifestyle changes. This understanding creates a long-lasting partnership between the provider and receiver of the service that contributes towards positive outcomes.

The literature (Barth, van der Meer, Hoepelman, Schrooders, et al., 2008; Barth, Tempelman, Smelt, Wensing, et al., subm.; see Barth, 2010) teaches us that chronic disease management and long-term compliance are very difficult to maintain. Although we recognise the responsibilities of both partners, it is still the provider who has to initiate motivational programmes and other control measures to assist the client with his/her compliance.

NCG introduced an intensive adherence management system into its chronic disease management programmes to this effect, especially the TB and HAART programmes. We have the opportunity to introduce this also for other chronic ailments.

Adherence management starts with primary and secondary prevention. It needs to be an integral part of all programmes. All clients who show symptoms and signs of early disease have to be made aware that they will eventually end up in a treatment programme. NCG designed the coaching of those clients in such a way that morbidity and mortality remain restricted to a minimum.

Once the patients are entered in treatment programmes, adherence management becomes part of the treatment management:

— *Adherence to scheduled visits:*

Patients are monitored about attending their visits on the scheduled dates. If patients do not turn up within three days of their planned visit, they are flagged and followed up. They are contacted by telephone, or a home visit will be made if the patients do not respond.

— *Pill counts and/or treatment compliance:*

Each clinic visit starts with the counsellor, and at each visit attention is paid to compliance through pill counts. Questionnaire feedback from the patient is requested about treatment issues, which pill is taken how many times a day, issues like at what times the treatment is taken, and whether they experience any problems.

— *Laboratory monitoring:*

Regular laboratory monitoring can provide important data about therapy compliance. In the case of HIV, the viral load, CD4 count, haematology and chemistry can provide important information around compliance, treatment regime failure, side effects of the ART regime, etc. Regular laboratory monitoring is not only important for the individual disease monitoring but also for cohort management, resistance development (Barth, Wensing, Tempelman, et al. 2008), and the evaluation of long-term results of rollout programmes. Laboratory results are plotted on graphs to illustrate the progress for the patient as a motivator for compliance.

– *Step-up Adherence Programme:*
This is introduced when the above-mentioned measures show therapy compliance problems. Adequate steps need to be taken before disease progress, resistance development, virological failure, etc. become problematic. Indicators for step-up adherence management are:
  – patient indicates s/he is not compliant;
  – clinic visits show non-adherence;
  – pill counts show less than 90% compliance;
  – virological suppression is no longer present after previously being undetectable.
The Step-up Adherence Programme includes counselling the patient again, upgrading treatment knowledge, shortening the interval between clinic visits temporarily for intensive guidance and intensive diagnostic monitoring in order to improve adherence and treatment success.

– *Cross-referral of clients within the Rural Advancement Plan programmes:*
One of the main strengths of the NCG model is the possibility of cross-referral of clients amongst programmes that deliver consistent messaging and the proactive compliance management at all levels: sports, drama, music, youth clubs, home-based care, and life skills training in OVC programmes. The holistic approach of the Rural Advancement Plan creates moments of interaction with the individual, with the community at large or with a special target group.

4. Research Summary

4.1. Background

Programme analysis and outcome measurement have to demonstrate that all the measures taken also translate into better treatment outcomes. This analysis has been done within the framework of a dissertation (Barth, 2010). The study shows significant results.

Long-term virological data from sub-Saharan Africa is limited. Studies from non-urbanized areas and programmes with a long-term (2-4 years) outcome, including longitudinal virological data, are even scarcer. The outcomes of our programme are discussed here in the light of what we described above.

4.2. Research Objectives

An observational cohort study was carried out in a rural part of South Africa. Bi-annual monitoring, including HIV-RNA testing, was performed for all patients. The primary endpoint was patient retention. Virological suppression (HIV-RNA 1000 copies/mL) were secondary endpoints.

4.3. Data Collection and Analysis

A total of 735 patients was included in the analysis. The median duration of follow-up was three years. The patient retention rate at the end of follow-up was 65% (476/735). Substantial attrition was observed soon after treatment initiation (20% within three months). Relating this to an initial median CD4 of 68 cell/mm^3 and an average BMI of 19.8 kg/m^2 shows that patients come to the programme at a very late stage of their disease. More intensive and continued efforts in primary and secondary prevention therefore seem justified. A sustained virological response was observed in the majority of patients remaining in care. Some 549 patients (75% ITT, 94% mITT) achieved virological suppression with first-line ART. Suppression was established a median of 12 weeks after treatment initiation.

4.4. Main Results

Not achieving virological suppression was most often due to early attrition (134/186, 72% within three months after treatment start). Longitudinal virological monitoring showed continued virological control with first-line ART in most patients: 66%. Apart from a poor clinical status at baseline, male gender was independently associated with treatment failure.

4.5. Discussion

In this rural South African ART programme with access to viral load monitoring, good long-term virological outcomes were observed in spite of significant early attrition. Continued efforts are needed to enrol patients earlier into care. Furthermore, the observed viro-immunological dissociation emphasises the need to make HIV-RNA testing more widely available.

Another motivation for intensive, at least bi-annual virological monitoring is drug-resistance development: a major concern when treating HIV. The virus can select drug-resistant mutations in the presence of suboptimal drug levels. If ART use continues despite ongoing viral replication, accumulation of resistance can occur unobserved, creating long-term major problems for ARV roll-out programmes.

5. Conclusion

In his keynote address at the launch of the Comprehensive Rural Development Programme in Muyexe village in Limpopo (2009), President Jacob Zuma stated that being born in a rural area or the countryside should not condemn people to a life of poverty and underdevelopment. Our vision for the development of rural areas arises from the fact that people in the rural areas also have a right to basic necessities and the realisation of their potential and dreams.

In line with national and international strategies for integrated community development and health, the NCG 12-hour clinics contribute through:

- providing comprehensive decentralised primary healthcare services that address prevention at primary, secondary and tertiary levels;

- delivering services that are responsive to the community they serve and that retain clients in Rural Advancement Plan programmes for life;
- providing health services that are integrated with the National Strategic Plan and that serve the objectives of the District Health system;
- providing health services that are equitable, efficient, effective, and of high quality.

Notes

1. The WHO publication, Innovative Care for Chronic Conditions, building blocks for action, 2002, ISBN 9241590173http://www.primaryhealthcare.uct.ac.za/approach/whatis/whatis.htm
2. http://www.primaryhealthcare.uct.ac.za/approach/whatis/whatis.htm
3. www.mrc.ac.za
4. WHO report 2008, 'Global tuberculosis control - surveillance, planning, financing'. Available at http://www.who.int/tb/publications/global_report/2008/key_points/en/index.html
5. www.who.int
6. 'Mortality and causes of death in South Africa', 2005: Findings from death notification. P0309.3. Available at http://www.statssa.gov.za/publications/P03093/P030932005.pdf
7. Profile, South Africa, World Health Organisation, Available at http://www.who.int/globalatlas/ predefinedReports/TB/PDF_Files/zaf.pdf
8. City of Cape Town Health Services, Médecins Sans Frontières and the Infectious Diseases and Epidemiology Unit, School of Public Health and Family Medicine, University of Cape Town, 'Report on the Integration of TB and HIV Services in Ubuntu clinic (Site B), Khayelitsha' (Cape Town, November 2007), p. 2.
9. http://www.who.int/hiv/pub/tb/3is_mreport/en/print.html
10 Médecins Sans Frontières South Africa, the Department of Public Health at the University of Cape Town and the Provincial Administration of the Western Cape, South Africa, *Antiretroviral therapy in primary heath care: the experience of the Khayelitsha program in South Africa* (WHO, Geneva, 2003) p. 7.
11 whqlibdoc.who.int/hq/2002/WHO_NMC_CCH_02.01.pdf
12 Anti-tuberculosis Drug-Resistance in the World, Report no. 4, World Health Organisation, 2008.

References

Ali, M., Khalid, G.H. & Pirkani, G.S. (1998). Level of health education in patients with type II diabetes mellitus in Quetta. *Journal of Pakistan Medical Association, 48*(11), 334–336.

Asch, S.M., Sloss, E.M., Hogan, C., Brook, R.H. & Kravitz, R.L. (2000). Measuring underuse of necessary care among elderly Medicare beneficiaries using inpatient and outpatient claims. *JAMA, 284*(18), 2325–2333.

Barth, R.E. (2010), *Treating HIV in Rural South Africa: Successes and Challenges. Dissertation.* Utrecht: University Medical Centre Utrecht.

Barth, R.E., Tempelman, H.A., Moraba, R. & Hoepelman, A.I.M. (subm.). Long-term outcome of an HIV-treatment programme in rural Africa; viral suppression despite early mortality (subm.) In: R.E. Barth (2010), *Treating HIV in Rural South Africa: Successes and Challenges (Dissertation: pp. 83-94).* Utrecht: University Medical Centre Utrecht.

Barth, R., Van der Meer, J., Hoepelmam, A., Schrooders, P., Van de Vijver, D., Geelen, S. & Tempelman, H. (2008). Byond the clinical Trial: Effectiveness of Antiretroviral Therapy Administered by General Practitioners in Rural South Africa. In: A. Vermeer & H. Tempelman (Eds.),

Health Care in Rural South Africa: An Innovative Approach (pp. 263-274). Amsterdam: VU University Press.

Barth, R.E., Wensing, A.J.M., Tempelman, H.A., Morabe, R., Schuurman, R. & Hoepelman, A.I.M. (2008). Rapid accumulation of non-nucleoside reverse transcriptase inhibitor-associated resistance: evidence of transmitted resistance in rural South Africa; *AIDS, 22*, 2207-2217.

Benatar, S. (2004). Health care reform and the crisis of HIV and AIDS in South Africa. *New England Journal of Medicine, 351*(1), 82, 85, 89–90.

Blackwell, D.L., Hayward, M.D. & Crimmins, E.M. (2001). Does childhood health affect chronic morbidity in later life? *Social Science & Medicine, 52*(8), 1269–1284.

Bock, N., Jensen, P., Miller, B. & Nardell, E. (2007). Tuberculosis Infection Control in Resource-Limited Settings in the Era of Expanding HIV Care and Treatment. *Journal of Infectious Diseases, 196*, 108–113 (Supplement 1).

Buffat, J. (2000). Unemployment and health. *Review Medical Suisse Romande, 120*(4), 379–383.

Chernichovsky, D. & Meesook, O.A. (1986). Utilization of health services in Indonesia. *Social Science & Medicine, 23*(6), 611–620.

Cohen, D.(2000). *Poverty and HIV/AIDS in Sub-Saharan Africa*. SEPED Conference Paper Series, Number 2.

Dranga, H.M. (1997). Ageing and poverty in rural Kenya: community perception. *East African Medical Journal, 74*(10), 611–613.

Ensor, T. & San, P.B. (1996). Access and payment for health care: the poor of Northern Vietnam. *International Journal of Health Planning & Management, 11*(1), 69–83.

Gao, J., Tang, S., Tolhurst, R. & Rao, K. (2001). Changing access to health services in urban China: implications for equity. *Health Policy and Planning, 16*(3), 302–312.

Gandhi, N.R, Moll, A., Pawinski, R., Sturm, A.W., Lalloo, U., Zeller, K., Andrews, J. & Friedland, J. (2006). High Prevalence and Mortality from Extensively-Drug Resistant (XDR) TB in TB/HIV Coinfected Patients in Rural South Africa. *XVI International AIDS Conference, Toronto Canada*. Available at http://www.aids2006.org/PAG/Abstracts.aspx?AID=51350

Holman, H. & Lorig, K. (2000). Patients as partners in managing chronic disease. *British Medical Journal, 320*, 526–527.

Law, C.M., Egger, P., Dada, O., Delgado, H., Kylberg, E., Lavin, P., Tang, G.H., von Hertzen, H., Shiell, A.W. & Barker, D.J. (2001). Body size at birth and blood pressure among children in developing countries. *International Journal of Epidemiology, 30*(1), 52–7.

Law, C.M., de Swiet, M., Osmond, C., Fayers, P.M., Barker, D.J., Cruddas, A.M. & Fall, C.H. (1993). Initiation of hypertension in utero and its amplification throughout life. *British Medical Journal, 306*, 24–27.

Leyva-Flores, R., Kageyama, M.L. & Erviti-Erice, J. (2001). How people respond to illness in Mexico: self-care or medical care? *Health Policy and Planning, 57*(1), 15–26.

Ludermir, A.B. & Lewis, G. (2001). Links between social class and common mental disorders in Northeast Brazil. *Social Psychiatry and Psychiatric Epidemiology, 36*(3), 101–107.

Lynch, J.W., Kaplan, G.A. & Shema, S.J. (1997). Cumulative impact of sustained economic hardship on physical, cognitive, psychological, and social functioning. *New England Journal of Medicine, 337*(26), 1889–1895.

Marmot, M. & Bobak, M. (2000). International comparators and poverty and health in Europe. *British Medical Journal, 321*, 1124–1128.

Mengesha, Y.A. & Bekele, A. (1998). Relative chronic effects of different occupational dusts on respiratory indices and health of workers in three Ethiopian factories. *American Journal of Industrian Medicine, 34*(4), 373–380.

Narayan, D., Chambers, R., Shah, M. & Petesch, P. (2000). *Crying Out for Change*. New York: Oxford University Press for the World Bank.

Nyonator, F. & Kutzin, J. (1999). Health for some? The effects of user fees in the Volta Region of Ghana. *Health Policy and Planning, 14*(4), 329–341.

Power, S. (2008). "The AIDS rebel". *The New Yorker, 19 May 2003.* Available at www.newyorker.com/archive.

Robins, L.N., Locke, B.Z. & Regier, D.A. (1991). *An overview of psychiatric disorders in America.* New York: Free Press.

Stierle, F., Kaddar, M., Tchicaya, A. & Schmidt-Ehry, B. (1999). Indigence and access to health care in sub-Saharan Africa. *International Journal of Health Planning & Management, 14*(2), 81–105.

Tomatis, L. (2001). Inequalities in cancer risks. *Seminars in Oncology, 28*(2), 207–209.

Warden, J. (1998). Britain's new health policy recognises poverty as major cause of illness. *British Medical Journal, 316*, 493–495.

WHO-UNICEF (1978). *Declaration of Alma-Ata.* International Conference on Primary Health USSR, 6-12 September. 1978. The International Conference on Primary Health Care (PHC).

Zimmer, Z. & Amornsirisomboon, P. (2001). Socioeconomic status and health among older adults in Thailand: an examination using multiple indicators. *Social Science & Medicine, 52*(8), 1297–1311.

Part Three

Community Services, the Community Health Awareness Mobilisation & Prevention Programme (CHAMP)

Chapter 10

Community Services: The Community Health Awareness, Mobilization and Prevention (CHAMP) Programme

Sediko Rakolote[a], Mariette Slabbert[b]

Abstract

The Ndlovu Care Group operates in underserved rural areas in South Africa through community-based intervention programmes that promote the Community Health Awareness, Mobilization & Prevention (CHAMP) Programme principles. The NCG CHAMP Programme represents all the community care programmes in the NCG portfolio, and although community health (ATC) and community care (CHAMP) operate as separate divisions, the success of the Rural Advancement Plan (RAP) depends heavily on the quality of referrals and inter-service delivery amongst the programmes. The focus of this part of the book concerns the CHAMP plan and the programmes that support the CHAMP outcomes of prevention and motivation. The programmes that fall under CHAMP share a central monitoring and evaluation framework that underpins and aligns all RAP programmes.

1. Introduction

The 2007 Fact Sheet on Poverty in South Africa of the Human Science Research Council states that there are unique difficulties pertaining to comparative data in South Africa deriving mainly from the fact that, prior to 1994, a number of regions in the country – largely the poorest areas – were classified as *independent homelands* and therefore excluded from the country's data. New estimates of poverty from the same document show that the proportion of people living in poverty in South Africa has not changed significantly between 1996 and 2001 (UNAIDS, 2006, 2007). However, it indicates that those households living in poverty have sunk deeper into poverty, while the gap between rich and poor has widened.[1] In economics, the cycle of poverty, as defined in the Hutchinson encyclopaedia,[2] is the 'set of factors or events by which poverty, once started, is likely to continue unless there is outside intervention'. The cycle of poverty has been defined as a phenomenon where poor families become trapped in poverty for at least three generations. These families have either limited or no resources. Collectively, there are many disadvantages that work in a circular process, making it virtually impossible for individuals to break the cycle.

a. Senior Manager Ndlovu Community Services, NCG Ndlovu, Elandsdoorn, South Africa
b. COO Ndlovu Care Group, Groblersdal, South Africa

This occurs when poor people do not have the necessary resources to get out of poverty, such as financial capital, education, or connections. In other words, poverty-stricken individuals experience disadvantages as a result of their poverty, which in turn increases their poverty. This would mean that the poor remain poor throughout their lives. This cycle has also been referred to as a 'pattern' of behaviours and situations which cannot easily be changed.[3] The poverty cycle is usually called a 'development trap' when applied to countries (Valentine, 1968).

NCG wants firstly to advance rural communities through unpacking and addressing the absence of needs in a rural settlement in terms of normalisation of life. Secondly, NCG wants to identify and develop the talent and skills present in the community to improve the probability of career achievement and recognition and behavioural change through Asset-Based Community Development (ABCD).[7] The CHAMP Programme therefore isolates and addresses the factors in a rural society that:
− prevent normal participation and development;
− promote social exclusion and stigma;
− identify the enablers, barriers, and priorities towards normalisation of daily life;
− identify the enablers, barriers, and priorities towards mobilisation and development that will motivate the members of the society to achieve advancement despite poverty and adversity.

On entering a community, NCG appoints a community liaison officer who engages with the community at all levels and exploits opportunities to involve existing civil society organisations in the RAP programmes. When the community is ready, NCG conducts baseline measurements of the knowledge, awareness, perceptions and current practices within that community to establish what the specific community needs are. Once these factors are identified in a community, CHAMP teams can specify their respective primary[4] and secondary[5] targets and design a strategy or action plan to roll out the programmes. Outcomes of the different programmes are all measured and evaluated in terms of primary, secondary, and tertiary prevention and retention through motivation programmes, as described in Chapter 1. The overall objectives of CHAMP are aligned with the NCG aim of achieving rural advancement through behavioural change and improved satisfaction with life of residents of those areas.

1.1. CHAMP Prevention Programme

The NCG CHAMP Prevention Programme is a social marketing, screening and staging programme that mobilises the community towards testing for disease, creates awareness in the community around HIV & AIDS, TB, and risky behaviours, and destigmatizes the community's attitudes towards people living with AIDS (PLWA). The objective of the programme is to effect behavioural change towards less risky behaviour through primary and secondary prevention (UNAIDS & WHO, 2005).

1.2. CHAMP Children's Programme

The NCG CHAMP Children's Programme includes a range of services aimed at addressing prevention, screening & evaluation, intervention, and maintenance steps to promote normal development in kids and to develop existing talent and skills, up to the age they leave school. The NCG CHAMP Children's Programme also educates children who are traumatised through societal and other external influences to cope better and undergo the debriefing processes, and assists them to improve their personal and household circumstances in order to normalise their situation.

1.3. CHAMP Sport, Arts and Culture Programme

All NCG programmes create awareness and screen, train, and refer talented individuals to appropriate motivational programmes in the Sport, Arts & Culture programme. They are evaluated in terms of what they are good at and are then supported and nurtured with talent development and exposure to promote achievement and improve their chances of employment later in life. NCG CHAMP Sport, Arts & Culture activities also actively motivate clients in all the other NCG programmes to remain in NCG programmes. It is often difficult to captivate people's attention in learning programmes and developmental activities unless the programmes are entertaining and fun. This component of CHAMP facilitates 'Retention through motivation'.

1.4. CHAMP Community Involvement

The Community Involvement Programme identifies infrastructure deficiencies in essential services and commercial opportunities present in the community, and addresses them through the development and stimulation of:
— Entrepreneurship: development of small and medium-sized enterprises that benefit the employees or the community. Examples are the bakery and car wash.
— Water programmes: drill and equip communal water supply points in the most needed areas within our target area and hand them over to the community water forums.
— Waste project: refuse removal in the residential area from strategically placed waste dumps.

1.5. Community Liaison

A full-time community liaison officer engages with the communities to obtain community participation at all levels before NCG embarks on new initiatives to ensure community involvement and acceptance for the new programmes.

Collectively, the Community Development Programmes empower people with knowledge on health and social issues, and provide service facilities to improve daily living in the rural communities they serve. This drive rests on the belief that individual awareness leads to community mobilisation, which in turn leads to social inclusion and achievement at individual, family, and community levels.[6]

2. What is Community Development?

The Merriam-Webster dictionary defines the term *community* as a group of people with common interests who live in a particular area or an interacting population of various kinds of individuals in a common location. The same source describes *development* as a holistic and participatory process that leads to growth, which is premised on the improvement of the standard of living of the identified groups. This is usually carried out through the transformation of power relations, the enhancement of capacity, and the improvement of access to goods and services.

It is difficult to arrive at a single common definition of successful community development; this task is always fraught with contestations (De Beer & Swanepoel, 2005). This attests to the divergent views on what communities need (Barraket, 2001). On the one hand, community development can be defined as a practice of civic leaders, activists, citizens and professionals involved in the improvement of a variety of facets of local communities. It can also be viewed as the process of building local economies while developing the community's capacity for self-driven and directed development as well as strengthening social ties. All these principles address what goes into developing communities. NCG's definition of community development is adopted from the broader context of the mandate of the Department of Social Development and the government of South Africa. In this context, community development is the process and method aimed at enhancing the capacity of communities to respond to their own needs, through community mobilisation, strength-based approaches and empowerment (Draft Community Development Policy of Department of Social Development, 2009). This definition puts emphasis on the participation of communities in their own development, and the mobilisation and provision of resources based on community initiatives. CHAMP expands the national strategy with the concept of ABCD, which identifies and develops assets and talents that are already present in the community rather than obtaining help from outside institutions.

3. CHAMP Role in Rural Community Development

The NCG CHAMP Programme provides a society with a future orientation, through social transformation and individual achievement. CHAMP wants to achieve measurable behavioural change and improved satisfaction with life in the target communities through a three-factor approach:
- Awareness, Education, and Information that encourages behavioural change in individuals, families and communities.
- Normalisation of daily life by addressing the absence of basic human needs with services and social exclusion through destigmatization.
- Mobilisation of individuals towards actualisation by identifying and developing community talents and skills already present (ABCD), to motivate and enforce changed behaviour.

Asset-based community development can be defined as follows.[7] It is an approach to community development which advocates the utilisation of the positive aspects present within the community, rather than focusing on the negative aspects. It puts the people who live in the community at the centre of community development. '*Individuals* should be the focus of anything that is done, and every person has skills, talents, gifts and passions that can be used for the community if they were known and the person was asked if s/he would be willing to use them.' People are asked to complete a questionnaire that begins the process of surveying what the community is good at, what they would be willing to teach, and what they would be willing to learn.

The second area that ABCD focuses on is the *associations* that exist in every single community. The website defines an association as any group of people who come together because of a shared interest or because of a common cause. Even the poorest or most remote settlements use associations for organizing the community. Examples include the churches, labour unions, social athletic clubs, political parties, or fraternal organizations. These associations of people already exist and should be utilized as platforms for advocacy and social marketing. The third area that is important to a community covers the *institutions* that support a specific community. They could be businesses, local government, large and small non-profit organizations, schools, hospitals, libraries, etc. All of these institutions could have space, expertise, buying power, employment prospects and many more great opportunities that are a strong asset to a local community.

The adverse economic and social conditions in the targeted rural areas where NCG operates require major upliftment projects at the community level. The idea of sustainable development is that the communities themselves, with appropriate assistance, must acquire the capacity to implement and maintain economic and social programmes. Rural areas face major challenges involving poverty, unemployment, HIV & AIDS, and the absence of essential household services. The government alone cannot cope with the developmental demand in rural South Africa. Proactive societal involvement is needed to support the government in its task (Rehle, Shisana, Pillay et al., 2007).

NCG as a non-governmental organization (NGO) has enormous potential to contribute positively to the development of targeted communities, as it attempts to change the communities from the inside out, rather than from the top down. Some of the positive attributes of operating as a hands-on NGO within the community are that:
- NCG has a 16-year track record of community intervention programmes that deliver the desired results;
- NCG actively initiates direct contact and communication with the community;
- NCG has the ability and capacity to innovate and adapt to changing environments;
- NCG works in those areas with very limited access to services and therefore reaches the most vulnerable and the most needy.

The NCG CHAMP Programme has been designed to target people along a continuum of care involving primary, secondary and tertiary prevention, and retention in programmes through motivation. CHAMP is focused on providing access to a nor-

malised environment that includes the housing, healthcare, food, water and social security that are guaranteed by the Constitution, with a specific focus on addressing the needs of:
- orphaned and vulnerable children;
- people living with HIV/AIDS; and
- unemployed people.

The CHAMP Programme objectives are aligned to attempt to achieve the following Millennium Development Goals at the community level:

- Eradicate extreme poverty and hunger
- Achieve universal primary education
- Promote gender equality and empower women
- Combat HIV/AIDS, malaria, etc.
- Ensure environment sustainability

NCG contributes towards these MDGs through partnerships with community associations, community institutions, relevant governmental departments, civil society organisations and active participation of the community involved.

Within the context of the NCG CHAMP, the different programmes:
- Deliver awareness and advocacy messages around prevention, destigmatization, and motivation that encourage community participation in the objectives and activities of the NCG CHAMP and RAP in general. These *Social Marketing programmes* seek to convince targets to reduce risky behaviour.
- Create social mobilization through generating public will by actively securing broad consensus and social commitment within civil society. Social mobilization seeks to convert knowledge into demonstrable action.
- Provide care and support to create an enabling environment for vulnerable groups and priority targeted groups.
- Achieve social inclusion related to the relative position of an individual or a group (a region) in the entirety of society. Each type of societal 'disadvantage' can cause social exclusion or inclusion, which is influenced by different social processes and dimensions of everyday life: economic, cultural, physical or mental disability, geographical (spatial), political and institutional. In other words, social exclusion is the outcome of a complex process and certainly not the result of poverty alone.

The success of community projects lies in the hands of the communities, but they do not always assume responsibility for their own development for different reasons. The CHAMP Programme involves communities in both the planning and execution of projects to increase acceptance and ownership. NGOs who are involved in community development projects need to realise that community participation is key to the success of all sustainable community projects.

4. Community Participation

Implementers of community projects often decide what the community needs on its behalf, without involving the members of the community and asking for their input. As a result, services are delivered based on just one perception of what the community's needs are. Involving the community produces better results through community ownership, and this increases the probability of sustainability and accountability. In some countries the notion of community participation has reappeared in discussions around the need to bring some local services and facilities more directly under the control of the local people. For example, the 2005 election manifesto for the British Labour Party argued for 'new opportunities for communities to assume greater responsibility or even ownership of community assets like village halls, community centres, libraries or recreational facilities' (Labour Party, 2005; p.105).

Experience in the field of community development shows that communities often understand their own problems and can often suggest innovative solutions if given the opportunity and the resources. Community involvement helps to deliver programmes which more accurately target local needs. Programme outputs which have been designed with the input from local residents are likely to last longer because the community takes pride in the achievement. Successful community development is not just delivering a product for its beneficiaries, it has to embrace social inclusion and the principles of ABCD:
- all communities have capacities that may not be obvious to outsiders, and it may take time to discover them;
- if it is to be inclusive, interventions and implementers must take into account different and sometimes negative ways in which the impacts will be experienced;
- flexibility is important, but this must not be at the expense of a loss of direction with regard to wider processes of social and economic transformation;
- capacity building is not 'doing development' on the cheap or against the clock, nor is it risk-free (Eade, 1997; p. 3).

5. Challenges of Involving Communities

Community development projects involving community participation are easier said than done. The potential for failure is large. The most common perhaps is that members of the community concerned are not genuinely involved and remain as passive partners in the process. The project is forced on the community, and as a result, the development activities are not sustained or followed up. The community returns to its old ways as soon as the project is considered delivered (Yusof, Batumalai, Wong & Okamura, 1989). Community interventions must not be damaging or confusing in themselves, and it is beneficial if they help to address poverty, early childhood development, safety, security, and ultimately a sense of belonging and actualisation, with the participation of the affected community.

Real community involvement involves compromises, sharing power, learning to cope with diversity, adjusting organizational cultures, understanding different styles of work, handling conflict constructively, and adjusting priorities and timetables. Communities may oppose projects when they are at first consulted about them, or excessive input can be received from inexperienced or ill-informed people, but with persistence, they can be overcome and real benefits achieved. In communities that have been marginalized for years, the confidence of local residents will often be low, and they might feel angry and frustrated and may oppose change unnecessarily.

Involving communities in partnerships requires time, resources and sensitivity. It is important for community leaders and decision-makers to be engaged and understand the purpose, scope and outcome of the project. Preferably, the engagement should take the form of informal private and not public meetings. Public meetings are powerful tools to inform the community at large and should be used after there is agreement with the community leaders about the aim and objective of the project. It is important that needs are mentioned spontaneously and that dialogue about the project is open and transparent. In NCG's experience, the relationship with the communities, and its community leaders, dramatically improves after appointing a dedicated community liaison officer.

6. Conclusion

In conclusion, the community development approach of NCG fully acknowledges that communities are capable of taking a lead in solving their own problems, with appropriate guidance, support, and mentoring. In avoiding what can be termed 'diplomatic colonization through donation', it is very important for donor agencies and organizations to respect the community's intellectual capacity in dealing with their own problems. There are challenges within communities, and one might be merely a lack of physical resources, but communities are definitely not incapable of solving their own problems. The people in a community were a community before the organization arrived, and they had various problems that they solved without external support, and they will always remain a community with or without NGO involvement.

We need communities to take a lead in dealing with their own challenges to ensure sustainable development through ownership. At NCG we believe that the community should take the lead and that we provide structure, support and guidance for their knowledge and skills.

NCG has a broker function between the donor and the community; NCG is in the community to listen to its needs, converts this with community involvement into a programme, and proposes it to the donor.

Notes

1. Statistics South Africa. (2007, 3rd July 2007). *Mid-year population estimates.* Retrieved 12th March 2008, from http://www.statssa.gov.za/publications/ P0302/P03022007.pdf
2. http://encyclopedia.farlex.com/Cycle+of+poverty, Hutchinson encyclopaedia
3. Hutchinson Encyclopedia, Cycle of poverty
4. Schools, Civil Society Organizations, Community at large
5. Teachers, parents, traditional healers, i.e. significant others
6. South African Department of Health Study. 2003. www.avert.org/safricastats
7. www.abcdinstitute.org

References

Barraket, J. (2001) *Building Sustainable Communities: Cooperative Solutions to Rural Renewal.* Sydney: Australian Centre for Cooperative Research and Development.

De Beer, F. & Swanepoel, H. (2005). *Community Development and Beyond: Issues Structures and Procedures.* Pretoria: J.L. van Schaik Publishers.

Draft Community Development Policy of Department of Social Development (2009). Pretoria: Government of South Africa.

Eade, D. (1997). Capacity Building: A People-Centred Approach to Development. Oxford: OXFAM, 1997.

Labour Party Manifesto 2005. Amazon.co.uk.

Rehle, T., Shisana, O., Pillay, V., Zuma, K., Puren, A., & Parker, W. (2007). National HIV incidence measures: new insights into the South African epidemic. *South Africa Medical Journal, 97,* 194-199.

Valentine, C. (1969). *A Culture and Poverty.* London: University of Chicago.

Yusof, K., Batumalai, S., Wong, Y.T. & Okamura, J. (1989). *The ABC's of community participation in primary health care.* Published by the Department of Obstetrics & Gynecology, Faculty of Medicine, University of Malaya.

UNAIDS. (2006). *South Africa: Country Situation Analysis.* Retrieved 14th March 2006, from http://www.unaids.org/en/Regions_Countries/Countries/southafrica.asp

UNAIDS. (2007). *South Africa: Country Situation Analysis.* Retrieved 22nd January 2008, from http://www.unaids.org/en/CountryResponses/Countries/south africa.asp

UNAIDS & WHO. (2005). *AIDS epidemic update: Special report on HIV prevention. December 2005.* Geneva, Switzerland: Joint United Nations Programme on HIV/AIDS (UNAIDS) and World Health Organization (WHO).

Chapter 11

The CHAMP Prevention Programme

Mariette Slabbert[a]

Abstract

The thesaurus[1] very aptly explains the task of a successful prevention programme aimed at behaviour change with the definition of 'convince': 'you convince someone to believe, but persuade someone to act, to convince is to get someone to think something, to persuade is to get someone to do something;...' We should be winning in HIV prevention. There are effective means to prevent every mode of transmission; political commitment on HIV has never been stronger; and financing for HIV programmes in low- and middle-income countries increased six-fold between 2001 and 2006. However, while attention to the epidemic has increased in recent years, particularly for treatment access, the effort to reduce HIV incidence is faltering (Global HIV Prevention Working Group, 2007). By 2015, it is estimated that there will be 60 million more new HIV infections around the world than in 2007 (idem). Sixty million more infections of a communicable disease that we know very well how to prevent. In an AMREF study, Mema Kwa Vijana conducted in Tanzania, which included knowledge, reported behaviour change and biological outcomes, only impact on knowledge and attitude was shown, with very little impact on reported sexual behaviour change and no real impact on any of the STIs or pregnancy rates[2]. This study highlights once again the difference between changing knowledge and changing actual risk-taking behaviour. With the CHAMP Prevention programme, NCG introduces a prevention programme with a theoretical framework drawing on theories and research from areas like psychology, sociology, health studies, marketing, and anthropology, which should result in risk-reducing and happiness-promoting behaviour change (Corrigan, 2000).

1. Introduction

According to Boler and Archer (2008) there are many reasons why interventions in schools have not shown the desired outcomes, including:
- lack of understanding of the factors which affect sexual behaviour, especially in different cultural contexts;
- structural barriers, such as poverty and gender inequality, which hamper behaviour change;

---

a. COO Ndlovu Care Group, Groblersdal, South Africa

– poor-quality and under-resourced educational institutions, undermining the quality provision of HIV & AIDS education;
– insufficient funding spent on equipping AIDS educators with the skills and resources they need;
– the pedagogical basis for HIV & AIDS education is weak;
– insufficient attention paid to international evidence of the characteristics of effective HIV education programmes; and
– fundamental disagreement on what messages about sexual behaviour should be delivered (in schools).[3]

The magnitude and seriousness of the global pandemic call for action (Bertozzi, Padian, Wegbreit et al., 2006). The appropriate mix and distribution of prevention and treatment interventions depend on the stage of the epidemic in a given country and the context in which it occurs. In the absence of firm data to guide programme objectives, national strategies may not accurately reflect the priorities dictated by the particular epidemic profile, resulting in highly inefficient investments in HIV & AIDS prevention and care. This waste undoubtedly exacerbates funding shortfalls and results in unnecessary HIV infections and premature deaths.

For an effective global prevention portfolio, we need to consider the design of 'prevention cocktails' that involve potent HIV-prevention measures for HIV-negatives as well as ones for HIV-positives (Fisher & Fisher, 1992). Worldwide, the vast majority of prevention programmes are focused on HIV-negatives only. Logic tells us that all new infections must involve a HIV-positive, so in order to effectively target HIV-positives to prevent more infections, prevention strategies should be aimed at increased uptake, and ideally 100%, of voluntary counselling and testing (VCT), followed by annual testing.

Fisher and Fisher (1992) presented a list of problems that most current prevention programmes are experiencing at the 2009 SA AIDS conference. Most prevention programmes:
– are a-theoretical and not informed by behaviour science models;
– do not assess their target groups, and therefore their programmes are not tailored to the target population;
– use messaging that is too broad and has a general focus, e.g. 'practice safer sex' rather than the more specific 'use a condom every time you have intercourse';
– provide information only, without practical advice on less risky alternatives;
– fail to motivate individuals and do not teach behaviour skills;
– are not rigorously evaluated;
– are not disseminated widely.

The UNAIDS annual report 2007, titled 'Knowing your epidemic', suggests that successful prevention programmes should involve so-called combination prevention. This strategy includes:
– addressing proximate (e.g. personal) and distal (e.g. environmental) factors;
– reducing infectivity and/or susceptibility;
– changing sexual behaviour and networking;
– reducing vulnerability and risk environments;

- focussing on short-, medium- and long-term impacts;
- scaling up complementary, quality, high-intensity and well-evaluated approaches based on emerging and proven impact;
- doing less of what has been shown not to have an impact;
- rigorous process and output monitoring and evaluation of results: outcomes and impacts.

The international community recognizes the urgency of stopping the AIDS epidemic, yet funding, political will, accountability and human resources have fallen short of needs. Although known interventions could prevent nearly two-thirds of new infections projected to occur in the near future, fewer than one in five people at high risk of infection have access to the most basic prevention services (Stover, Bertozzi, Gutierrez et al., 2006).

Prevention studies and national experience over the past 20 years strongly suggest that strategies are likely to be most effective when they are carefully tailored to the nature and stage of the epidemic in a specific country or community. Despite a limited amount of rigorous evaluation of prevention programmes, evidence demonstrates that tailoring prevention strategies to a region's epidemic profile is most effective and cost-effective (Askew & Berer, 2003; Bertozzi et al., 2006; Stover et al., 2006; UNAIDS, 2006; Wegbreit, Bertozzi, Demaria et al., 2006). South Africa's profile falls within the definition of *generalized high-level epidemics*, that is, an epidemic that occurs in regions where the HIV prevalence in the general population is 10% or greater and the highest prevalence in a key population, which includes sex workers, men who have sex with men (MSM) and IDUs, is 5% or greater.

The following activities are relevant across all epidemic profiles:
- surveillance of risk behaviours, sexually transmitted infections (STIs) and HIV;
- school-based sex education;
- peer-based programmes;
- information, education, and communication (IEC);
- STI screening and treatment;
- voluntary counselling and testing (VCT);
- harm reduction for intravenous drugs users (IDUs);
- condom promotion, distribution and social marketing;
- blood safety practices;
- prevention of mother-to-child transmission (PMTCT) and universal precautions.

Strategies that are advised specifically for this type of country profile should focus prevention programmes on broadly based, population-level interventions that can mobilize an entire society. Prevention should include:
- offering routine, universal VCT and STI screening and universal treatment;
- distributing condoms (male and female) free in all possible venues;
- providing VCT for couples seeking to have children;
- counselling pregnant women and new mothers to make informed choices for breastfeeding;
- implementing individual-level approaches to innovative mass strategies with accompanying evaluations of effectiveness;

- using the mass media as a tool for mobilizing society and changing social norms;
- using venues to reach large numbers of people for a range of interventions: work-places, transit venues, political rallies, schools, universities and military camps.

In a generalized high-level epidemic, contextual factors such as poverty and the fragility of the healthcare infrastructure will dramatically affect service provision at every level. The status of women becomes an overriding concern in this setting, requiring priority action to radically alter gender norms and reduce the economic, social, legal and physical vulnerability of girls and women[4].

The CHAMP Prevention programme, which is subsumed under the Community Service division of the Rural Advancement Plan (RAP), addresses primary and secondary prevention as described in Chapter 1 of this book. This programme was previously called the Ndlovu AIDS Awareness Programme. In 1998, NCG established its AIDS awareness programme as a community-based programme promoting STI, HIV and AIDS awareness in the community. It initially utilised social-cognitive models by Fishbein and colleagues (Fishbein, 1967; Fishbein, Middlestadt & Hitchcock, 1994). Language problems, a low level of literacy, and possible cultural bias amongst respondents were experienced because the measuring instruments, in particular questionnaires, were not translated into the native languages of the target groups and had hardly been socioculturally adapted. In this light NCG searched for theoretical models and measuring instruments adapted and suitable to achieve behaviour change in the communities it operates in.

At the end of the funding period 2005-2008, the Royal Netherlands Embassy (funder) requested NCG to perform an end of term review to determine the extent to which the set objectives were achieved. The aims of this evaluation were to assess the effectiveness, impact, relevance, and sustainability of the programme and to recommend changes that might be required to improve its implementation and outcomes. The evaluation made use of qualitative multiple methods of investigation including a brief document and literature review, in-depth interviews and focus group sessions.

In general, the consultants found the programme holistic and the integrated NCG approach unique in addressing awareness creation about HIV & AIDS. The review also stated that the team's mobility, interaction with other NCG programmes and external partners, and outreach work were keys to its success; they include theatre, entertainment, sports, and workshops as various means of reaching the community, and the use of information, education, and communication (IEC) materials and condom distribution.

Qualitatively, the evaluation confirmed that the interventions have led to an increase in awareness and knowledge related to the virus, its transmission, its prevention, HIV status, services offered by NCG, and caring for those infected. There has also been a reported change in attitudes regarding acceptance of personal status and of people living with HIV.

2. Target Groups

The CHAMP Prevention programme distinguishes primary and secondary target groups. Primary target groups are ones at high risk where we want to effect the behaviour change. Secondary target groups are those that will provide confirmation of the knowledge gained by the primary targets. For example, a school child (primary target) might receive the CHAMP message in class and will then confront a parent (secondary target) with the information. This parent might have cultural beliefs that clash with the message, leading to the child not changing behaviour based on the information from the parent. NCG will ensure that all messages are consistent and that both primary and secondary audiences are targeted.

The Prevention programme isolated the following target groups for its prevention efforts:
— Secondary schools (primary target) in Moutse East, Grade 9, training of core group members who will transfer knowledge within their own school environment (peer education) after the initial year to ensure sustainability and transferability of the intervention. Baselines are conducted with annual reports to principals that reflect the increase in learning and knowledge.
— Community (primary target): themed events that target men specifically to increase uptake in this group at workplaces, social venues, sport events, and community events; measurement will be the increase in the ratio of men who undergo VCT+ compared with the current male: female breakdown of 37:63.
— Civil society organisations: stakeholders (secondary target), local, provincial and national government, mentors, parents, teachers, traditional healers, faith-based organisations, etc. where members of the target groups mentioned above reflect on the message received from the prevention programme. Stigma reduction, utilisation of the baseline and follow-up surveys that guide messaging and programme content to improve social inclusion.

3. Aims

NCG wants to create champions in the community through behaviour change, achieve improved satisfaction with life, and deliver an effective communication campaign to achieve this.

NCG developed a social marketing campaign to uncover motivation and human behaviour in an attempt to convince the receivers of the messages to change their behaviour. The vision of the CHAMP Prevention programme is to 'Go MAD': Mobilise communities, create Awareness, and De-stigmatise the community members towards:
— increased uptake of voluntary counselling and testing (VCT+), TB testing, socio-economic screening, and childhood development screening and early detection;
— early care-seeking behaviour and staging in the appropriate RAP programmes to minimise future risk;
— early referral for treatment to avoid de-compensation;
— safer behaviours to support prevention efforts and minimise risk;

- effective inter-referral amongst NCG RAP programmes;
- openness and acceptance of people living with AIDS (PLWA), the poor and other judged conditions;
- gender equality & female empowerment.

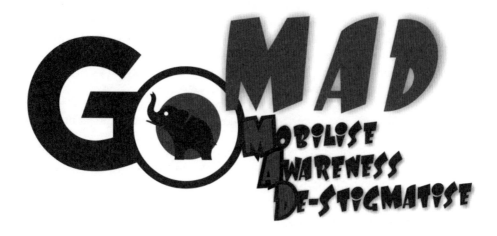

This takes place in all its target markets, with the aim of reducing the prevalence, incidence, and impact of the HIV & AIDS/TB epidemic and poverty-related burdens in the communities, and to improve satisfaction with life through changed behaviour.

4. Assessment of the Starting Position of the Target Groups

According to the same end of term review, the programme needed to address short-comings in the areas of monitoring and evaluation to demonstrate whether it is making progress towards achieving its objectives. NCG redesigned the entire pro-gramme, including its content, organogram and target markets, and repositioned the programme as the NCG CHAMP Prevention programme, rather than an awareness programme. The primary objectives of the prevention programme are to achieve be-haviour change in its target groups, and to improve satisfaction with life of the inha-bitants of the communities worked in.

Other direct recommendations to improve the effectiveness of the programme adopted include performing baseline studies before implementing new intervention programmes and sharpening the focus on specific target areas.

The fundamentals of the new prevention programme are:
- evidence-based interventions that measure behaviour change;
- outcomes-based activities that support the objectives of the programme;
- measurable outcomes that lead to rural advancement;
- a proper set of indicators to prove the programme works and to manage and monitor day-to-day operations.

When designing the new prevention strategy, the team debated at length on the question of why prevention strategies and community interventions to change behaviour fail or produce poor results, while the cellular phone industry managed to convince the whole of Africa to use cell phones within ten years. The answer lay in marketing strategies and proven models of influencing buying patterns. The team then queried whether it was possible to adapt and apply marketing and buying behaviour theories from the commercial advertising industry into a model for social mobilization that would result in more convincing messaging and behaviour change.

5. Working Methods

The CHAMP Prevention programme created a themed social marketing campaign based on the results of the knowledge, awareness, perception, and practice (KAPP) baseline study performed in 2009. The communication campaign strategy is based on the AIDA theory of buying behaviour that classifies the actions in the buying process into the stages of Awareness, Interest/information, Decision, and Action (Hoek, 1999).

The AIDA model of consumer behaviour traces the sequence of cognitive events leading to a purchase decision or other action; it is also called the hierarchy of readiness. Marketers use the AIDA model as a guideline for creating communications. This requires an understanding of where the market for a product currently lies on the AIDA continuum. Thus, advertising is thought to work and follow a certain sequence whereby the prospect is moved through a series of stages in succession from unawareness to the purchase of the product. Advertising cannot induce an immediate behaviour response; instead, a series of mental effects must occur with each stage fulfilled before progress to the next stage is possible. The premise of the model is that awareness alone is not enough to effect behaviour change. This can be illustrated by the following example: Should a person notice a new product like a cellular phone on the market, he would probably not go out and buy the phone immediately despite having the resources available to purchase the phone. Instead, that same person would first collect information on the new product from various sources like the media, friends who know about phones or technology, and other users. If these experts that he consults confirm that the intended purchase is a good idea, he would probably decide to make the purchase. If these experts advise against the purchase, the person would probably not make the purchase, or collect more information before taking action.

NCG believes that one of the differentiating factors in the success of this strategy lies in the fact that the programme delivers consistent messages to both the primary (the targeted group) and secondary (the experts or significant others that are consulted to confirm the message) target markets. The primary target market is described for our purposes as the audience that is targeted for behaviour change, e.g. schoolchildren. When the primary target, a pupil in this case, receives the message or information from the prevention team, s/he will test the message against a significant other that s/he believes has superior information on the subject. In this regard, the secondary target could be parents, teachers, peers or even traditional healers. The prevention programme engages with both sets of targets and delivers consistent messages to both groups. This strategy should also lead to destigmatisation as myths are replaced with accurate information.

The so-called new CHAMP Alphabetic Communication Campaign focuses on minimising the risk of HIV through awareness and promoting destigmatising behaviour. The campaign based its themes for prevention messaging on the following topics:
- Awareness creation, attitude change
- Behaviour change
- Convince; Condom usage, Circumcision, Counselling, Concurrent relationships, Child protection
- Destigmatise VCT+, HIV & AIDS, poverty and other stigmatised conditions
- Educate about prevention, illness & health
- Female empowerment
- Gender issues
- Healthy lifestyle
- Information on available support services
- Don't Judge PLWA and marginalised communities

The themes outlined above form the basis of all oral and visual training and awareness marketing materials of the programme. The programme uses billboards, t-shirts, radio slots, banners, and community events as communication channels. Effecting behaviour change is very challenging as HIV is deeply embedded in cultural, gender and socioeconomic issues. CHAMP Prevention programme messages are typically provocative and funky, and aimed at specific target groups.

The prevention programme not only creates mass awareness but improves knowledge that challenges personal and cultural beliefs through very direct, interactive, repetitive and personally relatable training and mobilisation programmes. The message is customised for the different target groups and is typically provocative. The mascots for the campaigns are animated male and female condoms called "'Dickie' and 'Fanni' a couple of Condoms".

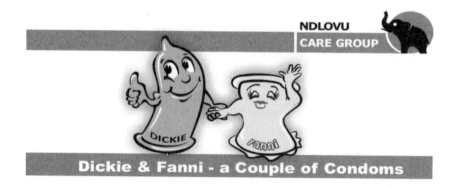

The 2010 FIFA World Cup campaign focuses on behaviour change and VCT+ uptake in men and is called the 'Men with balls' campaign. Typical messages include: "Men with Balls know their Status", "Men with Balls wear condoms", "Men with Balls are Circumcised", "Men with Balls respect Women", etc. The campaign targets men specifically and piggybacks on the upcoming soccer events and soccer heroes:

– Valentines campaign message for couples' counselling: 'Cool couples come at the same time' typically provoked discussion and raised awareness that disclosure between partners is cool.
– Domestic violence campaign: 'I am a woman. Not a sex toy. Stop women abuse' sends a very direct message when worn by women on a T-shirt.
– Messaging for schools: 'When you love her, use a cover', 'Dickie o chomee yaka' (Dickie (condom) is your best friend).
– NCG proposes that VCT+ is the entry point into the RAP care model, and VCT+ results determine whether individuals fall in the primary, secondary or tertiary prevention phase.

VCT+ refers to HIV counselling and testing that is immediately followed by a CD4 count to stage positive individuals at the time of testing, including TB questionnaire screening for early detection of underlying TB and, for women, a PAP smear for cervical cancer screening. Clients who test negative are motivated to return for annual testing. Staged individuals can be motivated with a referral, treatment, and care plan to stay in the NCG programmes. This practice improves patient adherence, patient compliance, and patient retention in NCG programmes. The CHAMP programme mainly involves itself in primary and secondary prevention and refers individuals to the Autonomous Treatment Centre (ATC) for tertiary prevention.

The CHAMP programme utilizes the RAP continuum of care, in line with the Herzberg two-factor theory and consistent with the levels of prevention, and retention through motivation, which enforces patient recruitment and retention in the RAP programmes:

1. Mobilise, Awareness, Destigmatise (Go MAD) campaign (primary prevention); this part utilizes the social marketing strategy to convince and persuade the targets in the population to prevent new infections through behaviour change.
2. Screening & Staging (primary & secondary prevention); screening targets 100% of the audience in the previous step to opt for VCT+ screening.
3. Referral into early care-seeking programmes (secondary prevention); patients whose diagnosis is detected early and who have a CD4 count above 350 are requested to return bi-annually for ongoing counselling and support and repeat CD4 count testing in order to monitor progress.
4. Retention of individuals in RAP programmes through motivation; skills building, support groups, entrepreneurial activities, and sports, art & culture programmes.

The CHAMP prevention programme achieves its targets through mobile teams that are specifically trained to address prevention and communication in a segmented group. The CHAMP prevention teams mirror its targets in demographics, age, experience, lifestyle, etc. to ensure their credibility. These specialist teams then develop activities, appropriate media channels, and messages to convince their target, under the guidance of external and internal trainers and experts. Communication channels often include role-play, dramas, public debate, SMS, movies, and music performances. Messages to primary targets: schools, community at large and civil society organisations (CSOs) are consistent with messages to secondary targets: significant others, including teachers, parents, traditional healers, elders, etc.

6. Evaluation

Measuring the success of a marketing campaign aimed at behaviour change is inherently difficult to measure.

6.1. In-House Monitoring Systems

Aspects of measurement are:
- The programme is compared within a logical framework that determines objectives, goals & projections, activities, outputs and outcomes for the different teams. The log-frame represents the annual workplan for the teams and the programmes as a whole.
- Operational systems that report as part of operations; these tools include daily, weekly and monthly tick sheets, monthly narrative and statistical reports.
- Quality assurance mechanisms that include flip charts and cue cards that standardise all the interventions and guarantee that the team delivers consistent messages.
- Quantitative baseline and progress indicators to measure the performance of the programmes against set targets and outcomes.
- Indicators to measure efficiency, effectiveness, and staff productivity.
- Set output targets based on evidence and historical data.
- Outcome indicators that measure achievement of Key Expected Results.

6.2. External Programme Management Monitoring Systems

The NCG CHAMP prevention programme works closely with different community structures (CSOs) and relevant stakeholders on raising awareness and delivering consistent messages. Part of the support that the prevention programme provides to these structures includes training, monitoring and evaluation capacity that allows the programme to measure progress against specific indicators and the achievement of objectives.

7. Organisation

The NCG CHAMP programme refers to and interacts with other programmes in both the community services and clinical services divisions in the RAP. Monitoring and evaluation also span across programmes as measures include number of internal referrals and the success of retaining clients in the programmes for life. For instance, the prevention programme performs VCT+ on clients and, depending on the outcome of the test, refers clients into the HAART programme, the wellness programme, the inpatient programme, or the different motivational programmes. NCG measures its success in terms of short-, medium- and long-term retention rates, viral response, immune response and resistance patterns.

The NCG CHAMP prevention programme cooperates and partners with community-based organisations, some governmental like the home-based care programme and some CSOs, e.g. traditional healers and faith-based organisations.

The Utrecht University, Department of Social and Behaviour Science, and the University of Pretoria, Department of Business Studies, are directly involved in the design, collection, analysis and interpretation of the baseline and follow-up studies performed on an ongoing basis.

8. Research Summary

Research carried out up to now concerned the former Ndlovu AIDS Awareness Programme.

8.1. Background

South Africa's attempts to prevent new HIV infections, as well as limiting the scaling-up of HIV care and treatment for the estimated millions of infected people, have shown the urgent need for an effective HIV & AIDS prevention intervention. Several research projects have been conducted to improve and develop the Ndlovu AIDS Awareness Programme (NAAP). Evidence-based results have provided NAAP with a broader vision to develop a more innovative and fun approach to reach many individuals and specific groups for AIDS awareness and Voluntary Counselling and Testing (VCT).

8.2 Research Objectives

Research objectives were:

(1) To evaluate the Ndlovu Aids Awareness Programme (NAAP); (2) to examine the cultural influences on sexual behaviour of participants of NAAP; (3) to determine the factors influencing participation in VCT; (4) to evaluate a tailor-made training on AIDS awareness resulting in a training manual for 'train the trainer' purposes.

8.3. Data Collection and Analysis

Several studies concerning NAAP are included. We assessed the study quality and extracted data from written articles. Interviews are conducted using self-developed questionnaires based on Ajzen's Model of Planned Behaviour (Ajzen, 1991). SPSS software was used for the statistical analysis. Several statistical tests were performed to measure the effects within NAAP. Logistic and linear multiple regression analysis, ANOVA, Chi-square and t-test were performed. Tests to compare and calculate differences between groups were done. Findings are expressed as β-coefficient and χ^2-coefficient together with their 90-95% confidence intervals.

8.4. Main Results

This summary includes four different study designs: pre-experimental, case-controlled design; one-shot design; a descriptive and explorative design; and a pre-post-test design. All studies are community-based and cross-sectional, and conducted in the Moutse area of South Africa. A significant knowledge increase was found after attending the programme more than once for both boys and girls. Of the sexually active children, 70.5% said they were willing to change their behaviour after attending the programme only once (Van der Lubbe, Schinnij, Tempelman et al., 2008). A significant decrease has often been shown in three beliefs after attending the programme twice or more: 'Having more girlfriends proves that you are a man', 'Sex with a virgin cures AIDS', and 'ARVs can cure AIDS' (idem, 2008). Abstinence seems to be an important means of protection among the respondents especially among the younger groups, and boys seem to be more sensitive to peer pressure than girls. Most adolescents who complete the traditional tribal initiation and circumcision school (IS) become sexually active because of the cultural belief that they have reached adulthood (Van Dijk, Van den Dries, Tempelman et al., 2008). More people plan to do VCT when they think other people whose opinion they value highly have a positive view on undergoing VCT. Men plan to do VCT in fewer weeks than women do, although more women than men actually undergo VCT. Older people were more likely to undergo VCT (Briët, Van Pelt, Greeve et al., 2008). An evaluation of a tailor-made training on AIDS awareness showed a small but significant improvement of pedagogical skills of the NAAP staff which should lead to more effective workshops, in order to ensure that students acquire crucial knowledge and change their attitudes and sexual behaviour (Rood, Van der Schaaf, Kanselaaar et al., 2008).

8.5. Authors' Suggestions

Further studies are needed to examine the actual behaviour change. In particular, a longitudinal research design is recommended to examine whether intention leads to actual seeking behaviour to undergo VCT and to evaluate the real effects of the programme (Briët, Van Pelt, Greeve et al., 2008). Paying more attention to reducing anxiety in men to get them to change their attitude about HIV & AIDS is suggested as a focus point (idem, 2008). Different approaches to sexual education for boys and girls are advised (Van Dijk, Van den Dries, Tempelman et al., 2008). Peer education appears to be of great importance with special attention to men, as men were found to be more negative about the opinion of valued friends and family than women (Briët, Van Pelt, Greeve et al., 2008). In future, the tailor-made training for the NAAP staff can be improved by combining the theoretical learning models with the practical part, and more information about pedagogical and coaching skills of NAAP staff should be collected by using observation materials and recording workshops (Rood, Van der Schaaf, Kanselaar et al., 2008).

Notes

1. http://thesaurus.reference.com/browse/convince
2. www.amref.org/docs/Impact%20Evaluation%20MEMA%20kwa%20Vijana.pdf
3. UK working group paper on the Abstinence Debate: Condoms, PEPFAR and ideology, 2007. Available from: www.aidsportal.org/repos/AbstinenceDebateEducationReport07.pdf
4. Fact Sheet #62E, Women's Global Health Imperative, UCSF; Nancy Padian, PhD; Stefano Bertozzi, PhD; Instituto Nacional de Salud Publica, Mexico, January 2007. Available from: http://www.caps.ucsf.edu/pubs/FS/pdf/internationalFS.pdf

References

Askew, I. & Berer, M. (2003). The contribution of sexual and reproductive health services to the fight against HIV & AIDS: A review. *Reproductive Health Matters,11,* 51–73.

Ajzen, I. (1991). The Theory of Planned Behaviour. *Organizational Behaviour and Human Decision Processes, 50,* 179-211.

Bertozzi, S., Padian, N., Wegbreit, J., DeMaria, L., Feldman, B., Gayle, H., Gold, J., Grant, R. & Isbell, M. (2006). HIV & AIDS Prevention and Treatment. In: *Disease Control Priorities in Developing Countries (2nd edition), pp. 331-369.* Washington DC: The International Bank for Reconstruction and Development / The World Bank.

Boler, T. & Archer, D. (2008). *The Politics of Prevention, A Global Crisis in AIDS and Education, p. 49.* London: Pluto Press.

Briët, L., Van Pelt, R., Greeve, F., Frencken, L., Van der Lubbe, K., Stroebe-Harrold, M. & Vermeer, A. (2008). Factors Influencing Participation in Voluntary Counselling and Testing: A Survey. In: Vermeer, A. & Tempelman, H. (Eds.), *Health care in rural South Africa: An innovative approach. Third edition. (pp. 201-229)* VU University Press, Amsterdam, the Netherlands.

Corrigan, J. (2000). The Satisfaction With Life Scale. *The Center for Outcome Measurement in Brain Injury.* Found At: http://www.tbims.org/combi/swls.

Fishbein, M. (1967). Attitude and the prediction of behaviour. In: M. Fishbein (Ed.), *Readings in Attitude Theory and Measurement* (pp. 477-492). New York: Wiley.

Fishbein, M., Middlestadt, S.E. & Hitchcock, P.J. (1994). Using information to change sexually transmitted disease-related behaviours. In: R.J. DiClemente & J.L. Peterson (Eds.). *Preventing AIDS: Theories and Methods of Behavioural Interventions* (pp. 61-78). New York: Plenum Press.

Fisher, J. & Fisher, W. (1992). Changing AIDS-Risk behavior. *Psychological bulletin, 111,* 455-474.

Global HIV Prevention Working Group (2007). *Bringing HIV Prevention to Scale: An Urgent Global Priority.* Found at: www.globalhivprevention.org/pdfs/PWG-HIV_prevention_report_FINAL.pdf

Hoek, J. (1999). Sponsorship: An Evaluation of Management Assumptions and Practices, *Marketing Bulletin, 10,* 1-10.

Rood, S., Van der Schaaf, M., Kanselaar, G., Van der Lubbe, K., Wubbels, T. & Vermeer, A. (2008). Evaluation of a Tailor-made Training on AIDS Awareness. In: Vermeer, A. & Tempelman, H. (Eds.), *Health care in rural South Africa: An innovative approach. Third edition. (pp. 225-249)* VU University Press, Amsterdam, the Netherlands.

Stover, J., Bertozzi, S., Gutierrez, J-P., Walker, N., Stanecki, K., Greener, R., et al. (2006). The global impact of scaling-up HIV/AIDS prevention programs in low- and middle-income countries. *Science 311,*1474-6.

UNAIDS (2006). Report on the global AIDS epidemic. Available from: www.unaids.org/en/HIV_-data/2006GlobalReport/default.asp

Van der Lubbe, K., Schinnij, M., Tempelman, H. & Vermeer, A. (2008). Evaluation of an AIDS Awareness Programme. In: Vermeer, A. & Tempelman, H. (Eds.), *Health care in rural South Africa: An innovative approach. Third edition. (pp. 159-173)* VU University Press, Amsterdam, the Netherlands.

Van Dijk, A., Van den Dries, H., Tempelman, H. & Vermeer, A. (2008). Cultural Influences on Sexual Behaviour of Participants in an AIDS Awareness Programme. In: Vermeer, A. & Tempelman, H. (Eds.), *Health care in rural South Africa: An innovative approach. Third edition. (pp. 175-199)* VU University Press, Amsterdam, the Netherlands.

Wegbreit, J., Bertozzi, S., Demaria, L., Padian, N. (2006). Effectiveness of HIV prevention strategies in resource-poor countries: tailoring the intervention to the context. *AIDS 20*,1217-1235.

Chapter 12

The Ndlovu CHAMP Children's Programme (NCCP)

Mariette Slabbert[a], Phinah Kodisang[b], Nthombi Mtshweni[c], Cheyne Neubert[d], Anke Gosling[e]

Abstract

The Ndlovu Care Group CHAMP Children's Programme (NCCP) targets vulnerable children within the family context and attempts to normalize their disturbed lives through the support of parents, caregivers, community health workers (CHW), child care committees (CCC) and partner home-based care (HBC) groups that are trained and enabled to provide quality services. Partnerships are also established with relevant government departments that assist with essential and basic services. The programme is developmental in nature, with the aim of mitigating the impact of HIV&AIDS, poverty, and deprivation on these children and their families in collaboration with various stakeholders on both a long-term and short-term basis. This is attained through raising awareness and mainstreaming of the Children's Programme into the civil society and the business community; networking and extensive marketing of the programme within and outside the country, and mobilisation of the community for support. The NCCP consists of the following programmes: (1) Orphans' Programme including the Child-Headed Households (CHH), (2) Nutritional Units and Pre-schools, (3) Life Skills Programme, (4) Dental Programme, and (5) Environmental Education Programme.

1. Introduction

With an estimated 5.5 million people living with HIV in South Africa, the AIDS epidemic is creating large numbers of children growing up without adult protection, nurturing, or financial support. Of South Africa's 18 million children, nearly 21% (about 3.8 million children) have lost one or both parents. More than 668,000 children have lost both parents, while 122,000 children are estimated to live in child-headed households. Whereas most orphaned and vulnerable children (OVC) live with and are cared for by a grandparent or a great-grandparent, others are forced to assume caregiver and provider roles. Without adequate protection and care, these

---

a. COO Ndlovu Care Group, Groblersdal, South Africa
b. M&E Manager Ndlovu Care Group, Groblersdal, South Africa
c. Manager Orphans and Vulnerable Children , Ndlovu Care Group, Elandsdoorn, South Africa
d. Manger Friends of Loskopdam, Ndlovu Care Group, Elandsdoorn, South Africa
e. Research Manager, Ndlovu Care Group, Groblersdal, South Africa

children are more susceptible to all forms of exploitation, increasing their risk of acquiring HIV infection.

In 2005, the South African government, through the Department of Social Development, issued a blueprint for OVC care in the form of a policy framework. The following year, it issued a national action plan for OVC. Both the framework and the action plan provide a clear path for addressing the social impacts of HIV and AIDS and for providing services to OVC, with a priority on family and community care, and with institutional care viewed as a last resort. The six key strategies of the action plan are:
1. Strengthen the capacity of families to care for OVC.
2. Mobilize community-based responses for care, support and protection of OVC.
3. Ensure that legislation, policy, and programmes are in place to protect the most vulnerable children.
4. Ensure access to essential services for OVC.
5. Increase awareness and advocacy regarding OVC issues.
6. Engage the business community to actively support OVC.

In recent years, political will and donor support have intensified South Africa's response to the HIV and AIDS epidemic and the growing numbers of OVC. The South African government has instituted guidelines and dedicated resources to create and promote a supportive environment in which OVC are holistically cared for, supported, and protected to grow and develop to their full potential. Government policies and services furthermore care for the needs of vulnerable children more broadly through such efforts as the provision of free health care for children under the age of five, free primary school education and social grants for guardians.

The NCCP is the result of a merger between the Ndlovu Nutritional Unit (NNU) Programme and the Ndlovu Orphans & Vulnerable Children (OVC) Project. The NNU Programme contributed experience with health, nutrition, education of guardians and community food gardens. The OVC Project contributed widespread community involvement and partnerships, success with educating the community on the Children's Social Grants, establishing a Life Skills curriculum for children, and education of guardians on issues relevant to the care and protection of OVC.

The impact of the HIV and AIDS pandemic on children is seen through the rising numbers of those orphaned by AIDS and those infected with HIV themselves. It is estimated that at least 1,765,167[1] of the 18 million children in South Africa have lost a parent to AIDS, and millions more are living in households in which one or more persons are ill or dying. In the absence of an extended family network, the responsibility of care and protection for surviving family members often falls upon the eldest child. The burden these 'child-carers' experience is multi-faceted and exacerbated by very little income and an under-resourced social network. In child-headed households, the biggest challenge is persistent hunger, followed by a range of other poverty-related concerns including: the struggle to pay school-fees; lack of school uniforms and other clothing; lack of money for transport and health care; inadequate housing; and insufficient heating (Streak, 2005).

While many OVC are taken care of by extended family and community networks, a rising number are required to take care of themselves and their ill parents/caregivers; and following the death of their family member(s), many children are left without a dedicated caregiver having been appointed. Although there are no figures to confirm how many children are living in child-headed households, estimates from the 2001 census have suggested the figure is anywhere between 100,000 to 235,000 households nationally (Proudlock, Dutschke, Jamieson et al., 2008). To support families and households caring for OVC, it is necessary to develop interventions "… ensuring that mechanisms are in place to provide psychosocial support to OVC and their families… [and to]…support skills training for child-headed households…"[2]

Infant mortality and malnutrition are major public health concerns in developing countries. In South Africa, infant mortality rates remain relatively high, with 45.2 deaths per 1000 live births and 61 per 1000 for children below the age of five years (Labadarios, Steyn, Mgijima & Dalda, 2005). There is an estimated prevalence of 8.3% for low birth weight. According to the National Food Consumption Survey (Steyn, Labadarios, Maunder et al., 2005), one in five children between the age of 1 and 9 years are stunted (21.6%), and one in ten children (10.3%) are underweight for their age. In 2005, within the project area, the prevalence of stunting was highest in children aged 1-3 years (24.4%) (Gardeniers, Klop, Tempelman et al., 2008).

The NCCP aligns its programming to the obligations laid out in international law and national policy frameworks in accordance with the following international conventions, goals, and other instruments that define the framework for action for OVC. Some key examples are listed below:

1. In September 1990, the World Declaration on the Survival, Protection, and Development of Children was agreed at the World Summit for Children. Signatories committed to a 10-point programme to protect the rights of children and to improve their lives.[3]

2. The Millennium Summit in September 2000 reaffirmed international commitment to working toward a world in which sustaining development and eliminating poverty have the highest priority. It also identified a number of Millennium Development Goals, some of which are relevant to the rights of all children, including OVC, in particular those related to education:
   - Universal primary education: by 2015, all children, boys and girls, are able to complete full primary schooling.
   - Achieve gender equality: girls and boys have equal access to all levels of education.

3. Article 26 of the Universal Declaration of Human Rights, which also deals with the right to education, states that:
   - Everyone has the right to education… Education shall be directed to the full development of the human personality and to the strengthening of respect for human rights and fundamental freedoms.
   - It shall promote understanding, tolerance and friendship… This right includes the right to receive HIV-related education, particularly regarding prevention and care. It is the state's obligation to ensure, in every cultural and religious tradition, that appropriate means are found so that effective HIV and AIDS information is included in educational programmes inside and outside schools.

4. The International Covenant on Economic, Social and Cultural Rights (1996) is the pre-eminent international treaty dedicated to the protection of economic and social rights. Article 9 recognizes the right of everyone to social security, and Article 11 recognizes the right to an adequate standard of living, including adequate food, clothing, and housing, and to the continuous improvement of living conditions.

5. The Convention on the Rights of the Child (CRC) is a framework that guides programmes for all children, including OVC. The four pillars of the CRC are:
   - The right to survival, development, and protection from abuse and neglect
   - The right to freedom from discrimination;
   - The right to have a voice and be listened to;
   - That the best interests of the child should be of primary consideration.

6. More recently, in June 2001, the UN General Assembly Special Session (UNGASS) Declaration of Commitment on HIV and AIDS set specific targets for all signatory nations. Recognizing that children orphaned and affected by HIV and AIDS need special assistance, nations must:
   - Develop by 2003 and implement by 2005 national policies and strategies to build and strengthen governmental, family and community capacities to provide a supportive environment for orphans and girls and boys infected and affected by HIV and AIDS by providing appropriate counselling and psychosocial support, ensuring their enrolment in school and access to shelter, good nutrition, health and social services on an equal basis with other children; and protecting orphans and vulnerable children from all forms of abuse, violence, exploitation, discrimination, trafficking and loss of inheritance.
   - Ensure non-discrimination and full and equal enjoyment of all human rights through the promotion of an active and visible policy of destigmatisation of children orphaned and made vulnerable by HIV/AIDS.
   - Urge the international community, particularly donor countries, civil society, as well as the private sector, to complement national activities effectively to support children orphaned or made vulnerable by HIV and AIDS in affected regions and in countries at high risk and to direct special assistance to sub-Saharan Africa.

Nationally, the OVC programmes are designed around the following key objectives:
1. Strengthen the protection and care of OVC within their extended families and communities.
2. Strengthen the economic coping capacities of families and communities.
3. Enhance the capacity of families and communities to respond to the psychosocial needs of orphans, vulnerable children, and their caregivers.
4. Link HIV and AIDS prevention activities, care, and support for people living with HIV and AIDS, and efforts to support orphans and other vulnerable children.
5. Focus on the most vulnerable children and communities, not only those orphaned by AIDS.
6. Pay particular attention to the roles of boys and girls and men and women, and address gender discrimination.
7. Ensure the full involvement of young people as part of the solution.

8. Strengthen schools and ensure access to education.
9. Reduce stigma and discrimination.
10. Accelerate learning and information exchange.
11. Strengthen partners and partnerships at all levels and build coalitions among key stakeholders.
12. Ensure that external support strengthens and does not undermine community initiative and motivation.

The communities of Moutse East and Bushbuck Ridge, like many underdeveloped rural areas, are entrapped in the vicious cycle of low literacy, high unemployment, poor job opportunities, poverty, and high rate of both medical and social pathologies and premature preventable deaths, in every age group. Overt development gaps such as poor housing, poor sanitation, lack of clean water, food insecurity, and serious backlog in service delivery, which impact negatively on the quality of lives, are rife in this area. The prevalence of HIV and AIDS and the escalating related morbidities and mortalities together with many chronic conditions such as hypertension and diabetes that claim many adult lives complicate the situation further, leaving behind many children who are orphaned, vulnerable, and often chronically ill.

Confronted with this situation, Ndlovu Care Group designed the Ndlovu CHAMP Children's Programme (NCCP) to meet the diverse needs of these children within the family context in line with the South African Children's Act (Act 36) of 2005, the Child Amendment Act of 2007, and the 2000 Millennium Development Goals. The programme started in 1996 with a nutrition component to respond to the pressing need of addressing chronic malnutrition-related morbidities and mortalities in children under five years old. The mobile Dental Services Programme followed this initiative in 2003 offering free dental care services and education to members of the community and primary school children. The OVC programme started in 2006, and the environmental education and awareness programme that promotes nature conservation and environmental care in primary schools started in 2008.

The NCCP covers a range of services aimed at addressing the prevention, early childhood development, social, intervention, environmental, and motivational needs of children to promote normal development in vulnerable children up to the age they leave school:
1. Nutritional Units and Pre-schools Programme;
2. OVC Programme including Child-Headed Households (CHH);
3. Dental Programme;
4. Environmental Education Programme (EEP);
5. Life Skills Programme.

2. The Three Waves of the HIV Epidemic[4]

HIV and AIDS were first identified in the early 1980s. Since then, the disease has spread around the world. Millions of people have been infected, and millions have died. This global epidemic ('pandemic') has especially affected economically poorer countries, particularly in sub-Saharan Africa. It has been described as having three 'waves':

- In the first wave, people are infected with the virus.
- In the second wave, people become ill.
- The third wave consists of the effects of people dying from HIV and AIDS, such as on surviving children and young people.

3. The Impact of the HIV Epidemic on Children

Many countries now have to cope with large numbers of children orphaned by HIV and AIDS. They will have to continue to do so for many years to come. Other children and young people, as well as orphans, lack support and are vulnerable to their environment. They include street children, children affected by conflict, disabled children, children affected by HIV and AIDS, and girls in general.

3.1. Orphans and Vulnerable Children

Compared to other children, orphans and other vulnerable children are more likely to:
- do badly in school and/or drop out;
- have poor educational and vocational opportunities;
- begin working at an early age;
- have poor health and nutrition;
- lose their rights to land and property;
- lack love, care and attention;
- experience stigma and discrimination;
- experience exploitation and abuse;
- suffer sexual abuse and exploitation;
- become HIV-infected;
- lack emotional support to deal with grief and trauma;
- experience long-term psychological problems;
- take drugs and other substances, and
- become involved in crime.

3.2. Resiliency of Children and Young People

Despite all these potential problems for orphans and vulnerable children (OVC), many children and young people show a great ability to cope, even under harsh circumstances. This is because the majority of children and young people are extremely resilient, particularly when supported by family and community members. Many families and communities are providing considerable levels of support to OVC in extremely difficult circumstances.

3.3. Supporting Family and Community Responses

Many people and organizations respond to this issue. There is growing evidence of what works and what does not. Orphanages and other institutions may seem a good idea at first. However, they are rarely an appropriate solution. They are very expensive. They can only ever care for a small percentage of all children in need. They often cater poorly for the psychosocial needs of children and young people, and they may undermine what families and communities are doing. The extended family and community are the front line in any response to children orphaned and made vulnerable by HIV and AIDS. Organizations seeking to work in this area should focus on initiatives that support family and community efforts.

The importance of this is summed up in five key strategies for work with orphans and other vulnerable children in the global strategic framework that was introduced in 2004. They are:

1. Strengthen the capacity of families to protect and care for OVC by prolonging the lives of parents and providing economic, psychosocial and other support.
2. Mobilise and support community-based responses.
3. Ensure access for OVC to essential services, including education, health care, birth registration and others.
4. Ensure that governments protect the most vulnerable children through improved policy and legislation and by channeling resources to families and communities.
5. Raise awareness at all levels through advocacy and social mobilization to create a supportive environment for children and families affected by HIV and AIDS.

3.4. Early Childhood Development (ECD)

Early childhood is the most rapid period of development in human life during which all children progress through a sequence of physical, cognitive, and emotional stages.

Neuroscientists have shown that the brain is almost completely developed by the time a child starts school (age 6). Young children respond best when caregivers use specific techniques designed to encourage and stimulate progress to the next level of development. ECD programmes improve young children's capacity to develop and learn.

Research has demonstrated that investment in all aspects of a child's development, health and welfare from birth to the age of 6 years has enormous long-term social benefits as it:

- increases the likelihood of children remaining in and progressing through school;
- reduces social and gender inequality;
- enhances children's later economic contribution to society;
- education investments at the ECD stage cost less than similar investments in adults and have more of an impact.

3.5. The Benefits of ECD Interventions

The benefits of the early childhood development (ECD) interventions are:

- Positive ECD programmes can change the development trajectory of children by the time they enter school. A child who is ready for school has less chance of repeating a grade, being placed in special education, or being a school drop-out.
- Children with quality early childhood education score higher on a range of competency measures when they go to school.

- Integrated programmes for young children can modify the effects of socio-economic and gender-related inequities, some of the most entrenched causes of poverty.
- A healthy cognitive and emotional development in the early years translates into tangible economic returns.
- Nobel laureate Heckmann (2000) argues that investments in children bring a higher rate of return than investments in low-skill adults.
- Africa has the youngest population in the world. Sub-Saharan Africa has 130 million children below the age of six years (20 percent of the region's total population).
- Although infant mortality declined to 105 per 1000 live births in 1997, it is still the highest in the world.
- Of the African children who survive to age six, nearly 30 million (one-quarter) are chronically malnourished, weighing only three-fourths of the weight standard for their age, due largely to inappropriate child-feeding practices, high morbidity and poorchild-caring practices.
- About 35 percent of children are irreversibly stunted because of persistent malnutrition before they reach the age of three.
- An entire generation of 130 million children below 6 years is physically and mentally ill-prepared for school in South Africa.
- In a society characterized by poverty, HIV and AIDS and the erosion of traditional family structures, investment in the survival and development of children aged 0-6 years is essential.
- Many adults in poor communities have limited knowledge about the importance of children's development, maternal health, nutrition, physical affection and responsiveness to their needs, and the importance of stimulation and learning through play.
- Children at home or with informal caregivers often lack adult attention and have limited access to educational toys and learning experiences outside their immediate environment.
- When impoverished children enter the formal schooling system, they are often physically, socially, cognitively, emotionally and spiritually under-developed; thus, they lack the foundation to begin literacy, numeracy and life skills work at school.
- Where formal childcare programmes do exist in poor communities, many caregivers have limited resources and training, and battle to deal with the children's needs and with the demands of the Grade R curriculum for 5/6-year-olds.
- In South Africa, only an estimated 16 percent of the 7 million children in the 0-6 years age group receive formal instruction during their pre-school years.
- A recent UNISA study (De Witt, Lessing & Lanyani, no year) in Grade R classrooms revealed that only 35.9 percent of South African pre-school learners have attained the minimum level of early literacy skills they need to proceed to Grade 1.

In line with the South African Children's Act (Act 36) of 2005 and the Child Amendment Act of 2007, the CHAMP Children's Programme wants to preserve and strengthen family structures and realise the following children's rights:

- family/parental care, or appropriate care when children are orphaned;
- access to social services; and
- protection from maltreatment, neglect, abuse or degradation.

The economic challenges of children affected by HIV and AIDS, and specifically children that grow up in child-headed households (CHHs) occur in four stages[5, 6]:

1. The first stage often begins when children realise that their parent has AIDS and is likely to die. They begin to fear for their future, wonder who will care for them, and worry about how they will be able to stay in school. Children are often pulled out of school to care for an ailing family member, or because meagre household income is now spent on the sick. School fees, notebooks, pencils become unaffordable, and children begin to struggle to provide care and replace lost adult labour and income.
2. At this stage, the quality of child rearing is compromised, and many important lessons on life skills and self-sufficiency are not taught, mostly because the parent is too ill to transfer the knowledge. After a parent dies, most children continue to live with the surviving parent or a relative, but often slide more deeply into poverty.
3. For some, the next stage begins when they find themselves the heads of households. A young adolescent may be responsible for as many as four siblings, some of which may include infants. Children who are the heads of households are in a difficult position not only because they must now support their siblings with little to no education and/or employable skills, but also because they most likely have limited resources. In many cases, much of the family's possessions may have been sold to care for the sick. Large numbers of orphaned children find themselves in homes that cannot afford to pay school expenses and drop out to work in the household, fields or on the street. Young children with minimal education or employable skills can be found doing work such as shining shoes, begging for money in the streets, bartending, selling food and, most often in the case of girls, becoming domestic workers (De Waal, 2002).
4. Many observers believe that the desperation of these young children makes them more vulnerable to abuse and exploitation, ultimately making them more susceptible to contracting HIV.

4. Target Groups

The Ndlovu Care Group CHAMP Children's Programme (NCCP) utilises various programmes that address the hierarchy of needs in children. On the one hand, to create a protective and supportive environment for growing up and on the other hand, to maximise the potential of the children to enhance their chances of freeing them from the developmental and poverty traps.

During the normalization of daily life, the NCCP addresses voids that exist because of the absence of certain basic requirements. The NCCP acts according to the definition of primary, secondary, and tertiary prevention and retention through motivation as described in Chapter 1. These interventions attempt to:

- *Primary prevention*: prevent these circumstances from occurring if they do not already exist.
- *Secondary prevention*: if these circumstances or illnesses already exist, then all efforts are aimed at:
  - detecting problems early, including developmental, health, psychosocial, dental, and economic aspects; and
  - assessing the extent of the problem and devising an individualised action plan to address it.
- *Tertiary prevention*: with an appropriate solution to the problems identified, prevent mortality and morbidity.
- *Retention* of the children in the programmes through motivation until they are old enough to graduate to an adult programme.

Several NCCP programmes address needs at these levels.

Orphans & Vulnerable Children

This programme identifies children who might become orphaned in the near future, children that are maternal, paternal, or double orphans, and children living in child-headed households. In the case of children living with dying parents: it is important to prepare the children and obtain birth certificates and other official documents before the parent(s) die, to mitigate the effects of family death and facilitate access to benefits, etc. The programme also identifies orphans and addresses their problems according to a needs assessment and database.

Pre-schools & Nutritional Units (NNUs)

The pre-schools enrol children before they start compulsory schooling, into either toddler or Grade R pre-school classes where their development is monitored according to WHO developmental indicators. Malnourished children and children that are referred from other Rural Advancement Plan (RAP) programmes (Clinical Services, Home-Based Carers, Life Skills or Prevention Programmes) are enrolled into the NNU with their caretaker for three months. The age of the children in the units ranges from six months to six years. The units provide identified children with three square meals per day, enrol the caregivers in a series of nutrition lectures, and assist the caregivers to set up a food garden at home. The children are brought back to health through adequate feeding and weekly doctor visits at Ndlovu Medical Centre, often receiving treatment for HIV and/or TB; meanwhile, the caregivers are empowered to properly feed and nourish their children, thereby preventing unintended abuse and neglect.

Dental Programme

A mobile dental consultation room visits primary schools and schools in the target area where they prevent dental decay at the primary, secondary, and tertiary levels. Dental awareness programmes teaches children about proper oral hygiene. Children are screened for dental and gum disease, and caries; these problems are staged and then followed up with the appropriate treatment regimens or referral for professional dental care.

Environmental Education Programme (EEP)

This programme exposes Grades R and Grade 6 children from schools in the target area to environmental education and conservation awareness in the nearby Loskop nature reserve. A camp to accommodate children overnight during weekends and school holidays will be completed soon. With no municipal services available to this community, pollution is a big problem in this area. Deforestation is another area of concern as most of the people living in this area do all their cooking with wood fires. This has resulted in a loss of most of the trees and plants in the area, which leads to soil erosion, which in turn can lead to houses collapsing, and poor sand roads. Another problem is 'water pollution'. Most houses do not have running water and need to collect water every day. If human or animal excrement or other wastes enter the water supply, the drinking water is contaminated, leading to sickness and/or death. The Environmental Education Programme provides tools and an understanding of why conservation is necessary, how to achieve and prevent loss while having fun at the same time.

Life Skills Programme

The Life Skills Programme arranges after-school activities and assistance with homework for school-going children in the area. The programme provides entertainment, social integration, debriefing, and academic stimulation. The programme includes a Saturday club that arranges sport tournaments and leisure activities.

5. Aims

The Ndlovu CHAMP Children's Programme (NCCP) addresses the plight of the orphans and vulnerable children in rural communities at five levels based on the Maslow[7] hierarchy of needs: (1) physiological, (2) safety & security, (3) sense of belonging, (4) self-esteem, (5) self-actualisation, and the Herzberg (1959) theory of motivation. RAP adapted Herzberg's two-factor theory for motivation in the workplace, and applies the theory to social transformation (see Chapter 1).

5.1. *Physiological and Safety & Security Needs*

These children lack almost every conceivable aspect of a normal life, ranging from protection against the elements, food, clothing, and nutrition, to the security of windows and lockable doors. At this level, the NCCP identifies the specific needs of individual households and addresses them. It is important that these children receive the basics to foster early childhood development, in an environment where they are cared for by adults, and ensure school attendance. In child-headed households, the biggest physiological challenges are persistent hunger, followed by a range of other poverty-related concerns, including the struggle to pay school-fees, lack of school uniforms and other clothing, lack of money for transport and health care, inadequate housing, and insufficient heating (Streak, 2005). Barriers to normal daily activities identified by the households include the following:

- Access to running water for washing and cooking; carrying water keeps children from relaxing, learning, playing, and developing. Boreholes closer to the identified dwellings help the OVC and other members of the population.
- Food: food security and household chores like cooking and cleaning take up valuable time in these households. NCG Nutritional Units identify malnourished children and enrol them for education, feeding, and day-care.
- Windows that can close and doors that can lock; security to protect against rape, theft, and sleep disturbance.
- Basic clothing, linen, blankets, school uniforms; social exclusion and stigma compromise these children further.
- Children are pressured to contribute financially to the household and turn to the streets to supplement lost wages, find refuge, and escape from stigma.
- On the street, children are exposed to rape, drug abuse, child labour[8], increasing the risk for contracting HIV.[9]

5.2. Sense of Belonging

Even children who are not HIV positive may find themselves rejected and alone. This only serves to add to the feelings of anger, sadness, and hopelessness that they may feel after witnessing their parents die slowly and painfully. One study in Kenya found that 77% of the children orphaned by AIDS said that they had no one outside of their families to 'tell their troubles to'.[10] The feeling of isolation can be heightened if the orphaned children are separated from their siblings, as often occurs when family members split up the child-rearing duties (Ayieko, 1998). Sibling separation can be difficult for children as they often rely on each other to cope with the loss of their parents. The NCCP identifies and adopts OVC as individuals, and then strives to create a 'family' support structure through the identification of informal 'foster' parents that assist with monitoring the children, reporting problems to the CHAMP employees, and social inclusion. This is a further effort to 'normalise' the daily lives of the children and to ease the burden on the heads of the families (child-carers). To support families and households caring for OVC, it is necessary to develop interventions.[11] Pre-school OVC need to be enrolled in the Ndlovu Pre-schools to enable heads of households to attend school.

5.3. Self-Esteem, Self-Actualisation & Mobilisation

The psychological impact of HIV and AIDS on children is often overlooked. Many children who live in heavily affected areas contend with the death of one or both parents, and frequently face the death of younger siblings, aunts, uncles and other relatives. Acquiring basic education and employable skills is an important part of preventing the spread of HIV and AIDS and breaking the cycle of poverty. Education has a number of positive impacts; not only are those who are educated more likely to have a higher income, studies have also shown that the educated are also less likely to contract HIV and tend to have children later in life.[12] The NCCP wants to see these children grow up and develop in a healthy way. Similarly, it wants to increase the probability of these children rising above poverty and illiteracy, through the identification of what the children are good at in music, sport, and education, and to support them with the development of talent and exposure to opportunity (Asset-Based Community Development). This set of developmental building blocks gives these children a voice, a face, and a future to fend for themselves.

6. Assessment of the Starting Position of the Target Group

The NCCP in Moutse currently has 3,500 children enrolled in its OVC programme. The programme runs a specialized Child-Headed Household (CHH) programme, under the OVC programme, that specifically identifies, screens, evaluates, and cares for children living in CCHs. The 3,500 total includes 80 CHHs that require intensive interventions, over and above the needs of other OVC, to ensure that they develop into productive and proud adults and parents. CHH that do not form part of the programme, because of stigma or social exclusion, form a special target group. The Dental Programme visits primary and secondary schools in Moutse, while children from the age of six months are enrolled into the NNUs and Pre-schools. The target for the Environmental Education Programme are 6-year-olds and 12-year-olds. The 6-year-old children are very impressionable, and if a passion for nature conservation can be fostered at this age, then their love for nature conservation grows over time. With the Grade 6 children, a more in-depth approach is used that is aligned with the school syllabus (see section 7.4). The idea is to create a passion at a young age and reinforce this with a follow-up in later years. More than 30 schools and 160,000 residents in Moutse benefit from the CHAMP Children's Programme and its activities.

7. Working Methods

7.1. Pre-Schools and Nutritional Units

The Pre-school and NNU project started with a nutritional unit next to Ndlovu 12-hour Community Health Centre, in Elandsdoorn (1996). Four more units have been established since, in Marapong (2001), Ntwane (2002), Thabakubedu (2004) and Phooko (2005). In each unit two community health workers (CHWs) offer training programmes to the caretakers and evaluate the malnourished children. These CHWs are recruited and trained from the local communities.

The NNU project establishes strong community-based care towards underprivileged, malnourished children. A maximum of 25 mothers/caretakers with their children are accommodated and trained per unit, three times a year. The pre-schools accommodate a total number of 300 children every year. These pre-schools monitor early childhood development, provide early childhood education to the children, and prevent malnourishment in the children and their siblings. The pre-schools run gardening projects where they harvest food for feeding the children attending the NNUs and pre-schools, and teach the caretakers how to maintain similar gardens at home.

The NNUs try to restore a normal feeding status as fast as possible to improve the well-being of the identified children, and educate caretakers to prevent disease and malnutrition in siblings.

Children in the programme are referred from other Rural Advancement Plan (RAP) programmes:
− children and their mothers who visit the 12-hour Community Health Centres;
− children screened during home visits by Community Health Worker (CHW)s;
− children referred from local and private clinics, and private doctors;
− children screened during home-to-home awareness days organised by the CHWs;
− children identified at community awareness events done in partnership with the prevention programme.

General practitioners at the community health centres screen the malnourished children, and the trained CHWs monitor them and perform the follow-up evaluations to ensure that the children stay healthy. The NNU project therefore bridges the gap between the doctors' recommendation and the caretakers' limitations in health knowledge.

The CHWs weigh the children weekly and check their development against a standard WHO first 5 years checklist. The doctor sees the children three times at the beginning of the admission and after discharge from the programme. The first consultation includes treatment for malnutrition, treatment for worms, testing for TB and HIV, and supplying medicines needed for a sick child. If necessary, children visit the doctors during the programme as well.

Staff offers all children HIV Counselling and Testing (HCT+) with the consent of a legal guardian. If a child tests HIV+, the HAART programme provides the child with medical care and Anti-Retroviral Treatment. If a caretaker refuses consent for the HCT, CHWs repeat the offer at a later stage during the programme. Due to the stigma of HIV and AIDS, not everybody consents to a HIV counselling and testing (HCT).

Malnourishment makes children more vulnerable to other diseases, and it is therefore crucial that caretakers are trained in related health topics, such as HIV and AIDS, TB, and other diseases. Besides information on different diseases, topics such as immunization, hygiene, safety, child abuse, and healthy foods form part of the caretaker-training programme.

A vegetable garden at home provides the whole family with the vegetables they need and even with a possibility to sell some vegetables to people in the community. CHWs teach water-saving methods and other low-cost techniques during home visits.

In practice, most caretakers need further assistance after the 3-month training programme. CHWs visit the participants at their homes after graduation and write short reports in the patient files. The objectives of these home visits are to inspect and assist with improvement of the home situation, and monitoring of discharged children. Every child and caretaker are scheduled for a home visit at least once a week, and discharged children are visited for two months to prevent relapse of the child and his/her home situation. The NNUs are located within the community to ensure access and adherence to the programmes. The coordinators and CHWs arrange door-to-door visits, to scan for malnourished children and to provide information on the impact of malnutrition on a child's health and development.

7.2. OVC Programme Including Child-Headed Households (CHHs)

Many of the children in rural areas find themselves living alone in grossly under-resourced child-headed, youth-headed, and elderly-headed households. Others live with sick parents or unknown relatives in extended families with no means of sub-sistence such as income, food, medical care, clothing, school uniform, family warmth, parental supervision, love, care and/or support. Many children are forced to drop out of school as they are relocated to distant families. Alternatively, they prematurely assume parental roles and engage in child labour to generate income, which is spent mainly on food and medical expenses of their sick, unemployed parents and family. Some children are caught in a web of social pathologies such as domestic violence, drug abuse, alcoholism, broken families, etc. and are forced to live in the streets, beg-ging for food and money to survive. In trying to escape their painful situation, some engage in self-destructive behaviour such as drug abuse, theft, alcohol abuse, and promiscuity, with resulting unwanted teenage pregnancies and HIV and AIDS infec-tions.

Some families get by on child support and old age benefits, while others find it difficult to access them due to the absence of official documents required to process the applications. The situation is aggravated by shortages of local public sector per-sonnel, resulting in delays in processing such applications, further disadvantaging deserving families.

In dealing with the short- and long-term effects of parental loss, and to normalize the lives of OVC, the Children's Programme:
- traces vulnerable children in the Moutse area and enrols them into a database;
- collects demographic and sociographic data;
- involves the Department of Home Affairs to arrange official documentation;
- involves the Department of Social Welfare, and assists with grant applications;
- supplies bereavement and debriefing support;
- screens the physical environment that the children live in, and addresses safety and security issues;
- provides food hampers to child-headed households;
- supplies school uniforms and clothing;
- refers children to other NCG RAP programmes that may benefit and motivate them, e.g. youth choir, music school, life skills programme, sport academy, envir-onmental awareness, and education.

7.3. Dental Programme

In the absence of oral health promotion and services in and around Moutse East, Ndlovu Care Group started the CHAMP Community Dental Care Project in January 2003. Oral health complements the holistic Rural Advancement Plan approach to-wards community health and community care in rural areas. The Dental Project pre-serves teeth and gums through awareness, screening, staging, and treatment, and promotes oral health and dental care for the children in Moutse schools. The target group includes children between the ages of seven and thirteen. Youngsters are eager to learn new habits, and their teeth can be preserved if problems are detected and treated early. These children are given a smile, a face, and a future through the delivery of decentralised oral health. The well-equipped mobile dental consulting room managed to see around 2000 children in 2008, of which 49% needed some form of treatment. Treatment includes preventative and curative dentistry.

During the school holidays, the community of Moutse receives oral health and dental care free of charge from the unit. It is sometimes difficult for the community to access public health services because of long queues and poor services. Almost all of the inhabitants appreciate the free service from professional visiting dentists, oral hygienists, and dental assistants. Pre-school children with dental problems are treated during the holidays; most of them are from the small village of Marapong where children have brown pitting marks on their teeth, which is caused by the drinking water in the area. Most of these youngsters with fluorosis experience social stigma. The dental programme addresses their plight with veneers built onto their front teeth that restore their confidence in public.

The dental team makes appointments with the different schools at different times depending on the number of children in each school. Starting with dental awareness workshops, where children are taken into the dental truck in groups for dental awareness education on how and how often to brush their teeth, flossing, and general oral and dental practice.

After the awareness education, the individual screening is done. Every child in a class undergoes a full check-up, and those with problems are referred to a special place for further consultancy. A form is filled out with all the necessary information and what needs to be done for the child. Then the forms are given to the class teacher to distribute to relevant pupils to obtain parental consent. A total number of 12,052 children were screened from 2003 till 2009 at schools, and 4997 dental problems were treated.

7.4. Environmental Education Programme

The philosopher Francis Bacon (1561-1626) expressed the paradox of man and nature neatly with the aphorism, "*we cannot command nature except by obeying her*". In his review of Darwin's book, *The Next Million Years*, Marson Bates (1954) states that mankind is a part of nature, subject to the force of gravitation, to the laws of energy transfer, to the need for food and reproduction. Yet, at the same time, mankind is separate from nature in the possession of the curious quality of awareness, of the ability to analyse and describe, to think, and to record and communicate thoughts. We can look at nature, study it, and change it in many ways. The CHAMP Environmental Education Programme (EEP) aims to create a society that will live in harmony with, respect and manage nature in the right manner. The children grow up and live in an area with limited basic services, and the EEP intermediary aims are to help improve these children's living conditions and supply them with tools to manage and enjoy nature in a symbiotic relationship. At an individual level, the programme wants to provide these children with the tools and motivation to work hand in hand with nature. Each child should walk away from the day's activities with knowledge that they can pass on to family members.

When visiting the reserve, each child receives a 12-page booklet on the following topics:
– the life cycle;
– herbivores, omnivores, and carnivores;
– teeth structures for all of the above;
– the importance of not polluting;
– reptiles;
– photosynthesis;
– general information about the reserve they are visiting; and
– the importance of trees.

Local taxis transport the children to the reserve. At the entrance of the reserve, all children board game-viewing vehicles and are transported to the Ndlovu Lapa in the reserve. An introduction to the day's programme follows, and the group splits into two: one group remains at the lapa for a lecture, while the other group starts on a game drive. Once they return from the game drive, both groups will sit down to a refreshing lunch and then swop activities. After both groups have completed both activities, all children visit the Loskop Reptile Park, just outside the reserve. At the Reptile Park, children see the different species of reptiles (crocodiles, tortoises, monitors, and snakes) and learn about the natural importance of these animals in our ecosystem.

All activities revolve around fun and include singing, dancing, games, interesting facts, offered by passionate facilitators, to ensure children remember the lessons learnt. EEP has two full-time FGASA (Field Guides Association of Southern Africa)-trained guides who ensure the children get the best education and are kept safe. The programmes follow the provincial Department of Education Grade 6 Natural Science curriculum to ensure that the children can implement their newly acquired skills back at school, and enhance their school marks.

The EEP runs four days a week, Monday to Thursday, 36 weeks of the year. Fridays are kept open to visit schools that have not yet joined the programme and for planning. The booklet also contains two projects that support the EEP activities that teachers can give to their children to complete.

Children and teachers are always very enthusiastic about attending the trips. The target groups are like sponges soaking up all the information relayed to them. The impact has been very positive, with the local reserve and reptile park reporting an increase in visits by local people from Moutse/Dennilton with the same children who attended the EEP outing. It seems that the children convinced their family members to take a trip to the nature reserve and reptile park, enhancing everyone's awareness and thoughts about nature conservation. When a school or child is identified by the EEP staff as being either orphaned, vulnerable or showing poor oral hygiene, the child will be referred to the appropriate Rural Advancement Plan programme to manage the problem. EEP works closely with MTPA (Mpumalanga Tourism & Parks Agency), previously known as MPB (Mpumalanga Parks Board). All EEP activities fall within one of their reserves.

7.5. Life Skills Programme

In her book on *Life skills: A resource book for facilitators*, Edna Rooth (2003) defines them as the skills necessary for successful living and learning. They are coping skills that can enhance the quality of life and prevent dysfunctional behaviour, and it is any skill that enables a person to interact meaningfully and successfully with the environment and with other people. Life skills are the competencies needed for effective living and participation in communities. The greater the range of skills that we possess, the more alternatives and opportunities are available to us, and as a result, there is more potential for meaningful and successful interaction.

As orphaned children lack parental guidance, the CHAMP Programme supports them with a psychosocial Life Skills Programme, designed to cater for learning needs, self-esteem building, developing coping skills while also assisting them with homework. Because of a shortage of funds, the programme is offered in only five villages with an enrolment of 250 children ranging in age from six to eighteen years.

Ndlovu Care Group trains unemployed youths from the township to act as facilitators of the programme; these life skills facilitators encourage the children to discover existing skills and aspects of skills needing development. The facilitators, or 'vochellis' as they are referred to in the CHAMP Programme, enable the acting out and rehearsal of skills through role-play, games, exploratory activities, group work, and reflection.

Orphaned children require intensive debriefing, for which the programme employs the 'hero book'[13] concept. These books are solution focused and can be used as a Psychosocial Support (PSS) mainstreaming tool in schools for example, as well as a focused intervention for more severely affected children. The hero book is a group-based approach and is therefore able to offer support to larger numbers of children in resource-scarce settings. 'Hero books' allow the child to decide on the challenge that he or she wants to address. There are numerous benefits to using these tools, they:
– are told in the children's own words;
– provide an opportunity for children to receive peer support;
– allow for normalization of problems;
– encourage sharing;
– can turn shame into pride;
– develop skills e.g. art, storytelling, basic counselling skills;
– build self-esteem;
– raise awareness of self and ability to express feelings and views;
– enable the child to be a hero to themselves and others;
– give children hope that change is possible;
– give children the opportunity to learn from each other's mistakes and experiences;
– provide a chance to move on from the past and focus on a positive life.

8. Evaluation

The NCCP uses appreciative inquiry[14] (AI) concepts to help focus the evaluation, and to develop and implement several data collection methods. AI was chosen as the main approach because it is a process that identifies 'the best' in a person and his/her work. In other words, applying AI in evaluation and research involves seeking out the best of what has been done in contrast to traditional evaluations and research where the subjects are judged on aspects of what is not working well. For this programme, AI was used to identify strengths (both known and unknown) in the NCCP and to identify and make explicit areas of good performance, in the hope that such performance can be continued or replicated.

AI workshops are held with programme staff, volunteers, and representatives from the South African Police Service (SAPS), and Departments of Social Services, Agriculture, Health and Education. In addition, educators, community members, guardians, and beneficiaries are interviewed to establish what they need from the programme, and observations of key programme activities are conducted. Visitors to the NNUs continuously evaluate how well the programmes run and pinpoint gaps in service delivery.

Ndlovu Care Group CHAMP Children's Programme has a comprehensive monitoring and evaluation (M&E) action plan. The plan has been designed to ensure:

1. that NCCP is doing the right thing in the right way and that its activities are producing real benefits for OVC;
2. that NCCP gathers high-quality data that can be used for strategic decision-making and improvement;
3. that NCCP makes the most efficient use of the resources available and that its programmes are relevant to the communities' needs.

Process indicators are continually reviewed, and staff measures targets they set for themselves. They also monitor the implementation of their activities. A baseline electronic tool has been developed for data-capturing purposes. Forms to identify OVC, to document services received, and record those not being serviced. The M&E Department provides ongoing support and consultation including data collection, data capturing and report compilation. To ensure the data are of high quality, regular feedback meetings are held where the performance is reviewed against targets.

Monitoring is an essential activity because it helps identify gaps, challenges, and OVC requirements, as well as ensuring that these needs are being met by the implementing partners. NCCP - through the M&E unit – will provide M&E training, too. Thus, by providing its partners with comprehensive M&E training, easy-to-use and up-to-date tools, NCCP is providing organisations at a grassroots level with important skills to make a positive impact on the lives of OVC.

9. Research Summary: Ndlovu Nutritional Unit Programme

9.1. Background

The limited information concerning the factors that determine the effectiveness of the nutritional programme on the health, functional and behavioural development of malnourished children and their caregivers has led to a number of research projects over the past years. Evidence-based results have provided the programme with more detailed information for improvement and expansion. This has led to a more comprehensive and holistic approach addressing not only malnourishment but all children's needs, to improve their health status and develop necessary social and emotional behavioural skills to cope better in life. The NNU Programme has been expanded into a Children's Programme focussing on the health, social and emotional well-being of OVC in the Moutse area.

9.2. Research Objectives

Current research objectives are:
1. to determine the effectiveness of the nutritional programme on the health, functional and behavioural development of malnourished children;
2. to evaluate the factors that affect the participation of caregivers in the educational part of the programme;
3. to determine the effectiveness of the educational part of the programme on the nutritional knowledge of the caregivers;
4. to develop a conceptual model of weight-for-age among children aged 1-8 years;
5. to determine the association between access to clean water and the risks of developing child malnutrition.

9.3. Data Collection and Analysis

All past studies concerning NNU were included; we assessed the study quality and extracted data from written articles. Interviews were conducted using self-developed questionnaires based on Ajzen's model of planned behaviour (Ajzen, 1991). SPSS software was used for statistical analysis. Logistic and linear multiple regression analysis, concept mapping and MANOVAs were performed. Chi-square and t-test were done to test significant levels (p). Findings are expressed as β-coefficient and odd ratios together with their 90-95% confidence intervals.

9.4. Main Results

This summary includes six pre-experimental, case-controlled and community-based studies conducted in the Moutse area of South Africa. An evaluation of the outcomes showed 57% of the malnourished children improved their weight above the 3rd percentile of the age growth curve after completion of the nutritional programme, and the majority evidenced no signs of relapse at an average of 10.5 months after being discharged from the programme (Westeneng, Okma, Veenstra et al., 2008). Caregivers following the educational programme score approximately 1 point higher on the knowledge scale of 1-10 than non-participants. These data show an increase in nutritional knowledge after joining the programme compared with caregivers who have never taken the programme (Klop, Gardeniers, Tempelman & Vermeer, 2008). Factors associated with an increased Weight for Age score (WAZ) are food availability and water source at a distance of more than 500 meters. Factors associated with a decreased WAZ are a greater number of children living in one household and the presence of infectious diseases. Income is positively and significantly associated with food availability (Klop, Gardeniers, Tempelman et al., 2008). The use of tap water as the main water source was associated with a 7.58-fold increased risk of being underweight after simultaneously adjusting for all the confounders, number of children in the household, immunization, and presence of waste on the premises. Children who lived in a house with water supply on the plot had a significantly higher score of wasting than children who lived further away from the water supply (Gardeniers, Klop, Tempelman et al., 2008).

9.5. Authors' Suggestions

Further studies are needed to examine the actual nutritional behaviour of the care-givers. In particular, pre- and post-surveys are recommended to evaluate the real effects of the programme on health, functional and behavioural development of the vulnerable children (Stofmeel, Wehmeijer, Tempelman et al., 2008). Of all the variables considered, water source was one of those most strongly associated with being underweight. Although the importance of water to child health is known, nutrition programmes should pay more attention to access to clean water as a potentially important preventive aspect of child undernutrition. Further research is advised into possible contamination of the tap water in this community and into the quality of tap water sources in general (Gardeniers, Klop, Tempelman et al., 2008).

Notes

1. Estimate made by Dept of Social Development when budgeting the National Action Plan for OVC in South Africa, July 2005
2. Strategic priority #1 of the *National Action Plan for Orphans and Other Children Made Vulnerable by HIV and Aids*, South Africa, 2006-2008
3. http://www.unicef.org/wsc/declare.htm
4. http://www.ovcsupport.net/sw464.asp
5. http://fpc.state.gov/documents/organization/32920.pdf
6. http://fpc.state.gov/documents/organization/32920.pdf
7. http://en.wikipedia.org/wiki/Abraham_Maslow
8. For more information on international child labour, see CRS Report RL31767, *Eliminating International Child Labour: U.S. and International Initiatives.*
9. Human Rights Watch, *In the Shadow of Death: HIV & AIDS and Children's Rights in Kenya.* June 2001. [http://www.hrw.org/reports/world/kenya-pubs.php]
10. Human Rights Watch, "In the Shadow of Death: HIV & AIDS and Children's Rights in Kenya." June 2001: Vol.13, No.4(A), p. 17. [http://www.hrw.org/reports/2001/kenya/]
11. Strategic Priority #1 of the *National Action Plan for Orphans and Other Children Made Vulnerable by HIV and Aids*, South Africa, 2006-2008
12. CRS OVC report for Congress
13. http://www.children-psychosocial-wellbeing.org/hero-books.html
14. Appreciative Inquiry is about the co-evolutionary search for the best in people, their organisations, and the relevant world around them. In its broadest focus, it involves systematic discovery of what gives "life" to a living system when it is most alive, most effective, and most constructively capable in economic, ecological, and human terms. AI involves, in a central way, the art and practice of asking questions that strengthen a system's capacity to apprehend, anticipate, and heighten positive potential (David Cooperrider of Case Western Reserve University, founder of Appreciative Inquiry; see e.g. Cooperrider & Whitney, 2005; Rogers & Fraser, 2003).

References

Ajzen, I. (1991). The Theory of Planned Behaviour. *Organizational Behaviour and Human Decision Processes, 50,* 179-211.

Ayieko, M.A. (1989). *From Single Parents to Child-Headed Households: The Case of Children Orphaned by AIDS in Kisumu and Siaya Districts. Study Paper No.7, pp. 7 and 14.* New York: UNDP [http://www.undp.org/hiv/publications/study/english/sp7e.htm]

Bates, M. (1954). Reviewed work: The Next Million Years by Charles G. Darwin. *American Anthropologist,* New Series, Vol. 56, No. 2, Part. 1. Apr. pg. 337.

Cooperrider, D. L. & Whitney, D. (2005). *Appreciative Inquiry: A Positive Revolution in Change.* San Francisco: Barrett-Koehler Publishers.

De Waal, A. (2002). "What AIDS Means in Famine." *The New York Times,* November 19, [http://www.nytimes.com].

De Witt, R., Lessing, L. & Lanyani, G.E. (no year). *Literacy and ECD fact sheet.* Pretoria: UNISA.

Gardeniers, A., Klop, E., Tempelman, H., Kuijper, L., Vermeer, A. & Doak, C. (2008). Tap Water Is Associated with Childhood Underweight in a Rural Area of South Africa. In: Vermeer, A. & Tempelman, H. (Eds.), *Health care in rural South Africa: An innovative approach. Third edition (pp. 115-124).* Amsterdam: VU University Press.

Heckman, J.J. (2000). Causal Parameters and Policy Analysis in Economics: A Twentieth Century Retrospective. *The Quarterly Journal of Economics, MIT Press, vol. 115*(1), 45-97.

Herzberg, F., Mausner, B. & Snyderman, B.(1959). *The motivation to work.* New York: Wiley.

Klop, E., Gardeniers, A., Tempelman, H. & Vermeer, A. (2008). Effects of a Nutritional Training on Nutritional Knowledge. In: Vermeer, A. & Tempelman, H. (Eds.), *Health care in rural South Africa: An innovative approach. Third edition (pp. 91-100).* Amsterdam: VU University Press.

Klop, E., Gardeniers, A., Tempelman, H., Doak, C., Vermeer, A. & Kuijper, L. (2008). A Conceptual Model for Weight-for-age among Children Aged 1-8 Years. In: Vermeer, A. & Tempelman, H. (Eds.), *Health care in rural South Africa: An innovative approach. Third edition (pp. 101- 114).* Amsterdam: VU University Press.

Labadarios, D., Steyn, N.P., Mgijima, C. & Dalda, N (2005). Review of the South African nutrition policy 1994-2002 and targets for 2007: achievements and challenges. *Nutrition, 21*(1), 100-1008..

Proudlock, P., Dutschke, M., Jamieson, L., Monson, J. & Smith, C. (Eds) (2008). *South African Child Gauge 2007/2008.* Cape Town: Children's Institute, University of Cape Town.

Rogers, P.J. & Fraser, D. (2003). Appreciating Appreciative Inquiry. *New Directions for Evaluation, 100,* 75-83.

Rooth, E. (2003). *Life skills: A resource book for facilitators.* Braamfontein: Nolwazi.

Steyn, N.P., Labadarios, D., Maunder, E., Nel, J., & Lombard, C. (2005). Secondary anthropometric data analysis of the National Food Consumption Survey in South Africa: the double burden. *Nutrition, 21*(1), 4-13.

Stofmeel, F., Wehmeijer, F., Tempelman, H., Van Aken, M. & Vermeer, A. (2008). Effects of a Nutrition on the Health and Development of Undernourished Children. In: Vermeer, A. & Tempelman, H. (Eds.), *Health care in rural South Africa: An innovative approach. Third edition (pp. 77-90.* Amsterdam: VU University Press.

Streak, J. (2005). *Government's Social Development Response to Children Made Vulnerable by HIV and AIDS: Identifying Gaps in Policy and Budgeting.* Pretoria/Cape Town: Children's Budget Unit, Budget Information Service, IDASA South Africa.

Vermeer, A., & Tempelman, H.A. (2008). *Health care in rural South Africa: An innovative approach. Third edition.* Amsterdam: VU University Press, Amsterdam.

Westeneng, M., Okma, A., Veenstra, J., Tempelman, H., & Vermeer, A. (2008). Evaluation of a Nutrition : Participation and Health Effects. In: Vermeer, A. & Tempelman, H. (Eds.), *Health care in rural South Africa: An innovative approach. Third edition (pp. 63-76).* Amsterdam: VU University Press.

De With, A., Wouters, M. & Jongmans, M. Influences on the Nutritional Status of Children (2008). In: Vermeer, A. & Tempelman, H. (Eds.), *Health care in rural South Africa: An innovative approach. Third edition (pp. 125-148).* Amsterdam: VU University Press.

Chapter 13

The CHAMP Motivation Programme: Sport, Art, Culture, and Academic Programmes

Mariette Slabbert[a]

> *'The greatest good you can do for another is not just share your riches, but to reveal to him his own.'* Benjamin Disraeli.[1]

Abstract

In the foreword to *Up and Out of Poverty*, the authors, Philip Kotler and Nancy Lee (2009), describe poverty as a chronic human condition, more like diabetes than polio, susceptible to external events and influenced by individual and community differences. The Rural Advancement Plan (RAP), explained in chapter 1, utilises a continuum of care that includes primary, secondary, and tertiary prevention programmes to deal with adverse conditions, and motivation programmes to retain people enrolled in developmental activities for life. This chapter describes the sport, art, culture, and academic programmes that through Asset-Based Community Development (ABCD) reveal the assets, abilities, and talents already available in rural communities and how they are utilised to assist these individuals to actualise their capabilities. Kotler and Lee state in the same source that the most pressing and fundamental need of the poor is hope, and that this hope becomes reality when the target segment of the extreme poor believes that the service provider has listened to them, understands the need, and has a planned implementation programme that will stay around to complete the job. They mention further that the poor are found at the local level and that "it is at the local level that ending poverty becomes a real possibility" (p. 43). It is specifically at the local level that Ndlovu Care Group operates and where it would like to contribute to the fight against poverty with the Rural Advancement Plan. The people from these rural communities and patients enrolled in chronic treatment programmes are made more vulnerable through poverty and other social and economic factors, including HIV & AIDS and TB. Through the Rural Advancement Plan, Ndlovu Care Group (NCG) wants to assist individuals in these communities by transferring business models for motivation (Herzberg, Mausner & Snyderman, 1959) and for buying behaviour[2] to the arena of social mobilisation and social marketing, to enable people to achieve more individually than they would achieve without the motivation programmes. The Rural Advancement Plan motivation programmes operate at the local level and rely on an understanding of the target

---

a. COO Ndlovu Care Group, Groblersdal, South Africa

audience's needs, wants, perceptions, preferences, values, and barriers, to turn this understanding into an effective plan to achieve desired behaviour outcomes.

1. Introduction

The United Nations formulated the Millennium Development Goals (United Nations, 2006) to significantly reduce poverty levels by 2015; of the eight goals, only one addresses income, the other seven deals with improving the human and social conditions of the poor. Stephen Smith (2005), in response to the book *The Fortune at the Bottom of the Pyramid* (Prahalad, 2005) points out that reaching the poor with products has not been the main difficulty. The problem is that before the extreme poor can consume anything, they need social capital, which consists of health, reduced infant mortality, protection from diseases, education to know how to use the assistance, and community connectivity. These are social and human development needs as opposed to dollar-denominated market needs.

South Africa is sitting on a 'social time bomb' with more than three million youths between the ages of 18 and 24 who don't have jobs and don't receive any education or training. According to a recent report titled *Responding to the educational needs of post-school youth* (CHET & FETI, 2009), it is not only an educational problem but part 'of a socio-economic disaster... Not only does it indicate a massive waste of talent, but also the possibility of serious disruption' (CHET & FETI, 2009; p. 13). The report states: "Unfavourable school and domestic environments influence black young adults' educational achievement and renders their individual abilities irrelevant." It also states that "the 'worst' thing that can happen to a student is to drop out of school between Grades 10-12" (CHET & FETI, 2009; p. 9).

According to the South African National HIV Prevalence, Incidence, Behaviour and Communication survey (Shisana, Rehle, Simbayi, et al., 2008), South Africa has the largest burden of HIV & AIDS and is currently implementing the largest antiretroviral treatment (ART) programme in the world. Adherence to treatment is a strong predictor of viral response in initial and subsequent antiretroviral regimens, and it is therefore of vital importance that patients initiated on therapy comply with the treatment schedules. According to the study 'Determinants of antiretroviral treatment adherence among patients with HIV and AIDS in Botswana' (Weiser, Wolf, Kebaabetswe, et al., 2002), to measure adherence (defined as taking 95% of prescribed doses) and to identify factors affecting adherence, the authors elicited patient knowledge, attitudes and practices; use of traditional medicines; structural barriers to treatment; and social stigma. The study found that the principal barriers to adherence included financial constraints (44%), stigma (15%), travel/migration (10%), side-effects (9%), and lack of food (7%). While 98% of patients demonstrated accurate knowledge about the mode of transmission and prevention of HIV, 70% of providers believed that lack of appropriate knowledge in programmes that achieve behaviour change (less risky behaviour) played a key role in the approach of non-adherence (Weiser et al., 2002). Eliminating cost as a barrier by logistical regression in the study increased the projected adherence from 54% to 74%. Because Ndlovu Care Group operates in the community through decentralised services, financial constraints and travel/migration effects are therefore mitigated, leaving behaviour change through effective campaigns to convince patients on treatment to comply. This study confirmed that awareness and knowledge alone do not result in the required adherence ratios (Weiser et al., 2002). CHAMP therefore initiates intensive counselling programmes for all enrolled patients to motivate retention and adherence. Trained counsellors conduct monthly sessions with patients; these sessions include screening for underlying psychosocial, economic and clinical conditions, and the message is underpinned with an academic framework to increase behaviour change. The counselling session also includes a pill count and a three-question adherence questionnaire to evaluate compliance. Results from the counselling evaluation determine whether counselling therapy is stepped up or whether referral to specialists and support are required. Standardised tools ensure that counsellors do not stray from accurate knowledge and that they cover all aspects of a counselling area (see Chapter 7).

Kotler and Lee (2009) state that "Marketing, properly applied, goes beyond the important contribution of Prahalad, who has promoted meeting the wants of the poor as a profit opportunity; social marketing programmes sell behaviours to typically influence target audiences to do four things, also referred to as the main principles of social marketing:
- accept a new behaviour (mosquito net);
- reject a potentially undesirable behaviour (start to smoke);
- modify a current behaviour (*consistent* condom use); and
- abandon an old, undesirable behaviour (excessive alcohol use)" (Kotler & Lee, 2009; p. 56).

According to Kotler & Lee (2009), the bottom line is that the target should buy into the new behaviour that the social marketing programme sells. It is therefore necessary to gain insight into how the *customer* perceives the *cost* of changing their behaviour and situation. It poses the question of what can tip the balance in favour of poverty-escaping behaviour.

Martin Seligman speculates in his book *Authentic Happiness* (2003) that people who are impoverished, depressed, or suicidal care about much more than the relief of their suffering. These persons care – sometimes desperately – about virtue, about purpose, about integrity, and about meaning. Experiences that induce positive emotions cause negative emotions to dissipate rapidly. The strengths and virtues function to buffer against misfortune and against the psychological disorders, and they may be the key to building resilience. The best therapists do not merely heal damage, they help people identify and build their strengths and their virtues. Seligman explains that positive emotions about the future include faith, trust, confidence, hope, and optimism.

The Ndlovu Care Group sport, arts and culture programmes express a collective culture embracing behaviours, habits, language, art, craft, music, dance, drama, literature, customs, religions, work, social occasions, recreation and the total way of life. Through art and culture, heritage is handed down to future generations. Key characteristics are:

- Arts and culture activities are essential to the health and well-being of society. They should be available to all citizens, regardless of circumstance, income or ethnic origin.
- The artistic and cultural life of the community is a central feature of its character and identity, and it attracts permanent residents and visitors to the community.
- The benefits of an active artistic and cultural life permeate all sections of the community.
- A vigorous arts and cultural programme enriches the lives of people in the community, whilst creating opportunities for enterprise and employment.

The principles of the programme are:
- Accessibility: removing barriers, providing opportunity for all arts and cultural groups / individuals in the community.
- Diversity: accommodating lifestyles, ethnicity and culture of the individuals in the community.
- Sustainability: meeting the needs of the present without compromising the ability of future generations to meet their own needs.
- Prosperity: providing abundance of opportunities.
- Partnerships: develop and sustain partnerships that are open, honest, and undertaken with integrity.

The CHAMP motivation programmes utilise various interventions that address the hierarchy of needs and wants in rural populations to maximise the potential of these individuals and to enhance their chances of creating a better future for themselves and their communities. When introducing community development and chronic treatment programmes, these interventions usually appear to be successful at motivating individuals to initiate goal pursuits, but they rarely address the real problem with adherence and compliance, and that is goal maintenance (Rothman, 2000). One of the main objectives of the Rural Advancement Plan is to retain individuals in community programmes for life, through motivation. The Rural Advancement Plan suggests that by drawing on theories and research from areas like psychology, sociology, health studies, and anthropology, it is possible to devise risk-reducing and happiness-promoting behavioural change. It is important that community interventions are not damaging or confusing in themselves, and it is beneficial if they help to address poverty, early childhood development, safety, security, and ultimately sense of belonging and actualisation, in collaboration with the community. The Rural Advancement Plan motivates individuals and subsequently supports rural communities through services that enhance self-esteem, actualisation, well-being and freedom. In other words, as well as improving matters for people in rural areas, by addressing unpleasantness and difficulties, community development workers must aim to enhance well-being at three different levels: (1) sense of belonging (family life and support structures), (2) self-esteem, and (3) self-actualisation.

Removing discomfort has to be worthwhile (through addressing the absence of things) and has to motivate the individual to move to the next level, closer to the higher-order needs.

The CHAMP motivation programme equips talented people with additional skills and attitudes supportive of developing successful futures. Developing their life skills involves covering all the aspects of development that result in optimum health, proper education, and positive overall outcomes. To this end, singing, music, sport, art and other cultural activities are used.

Although South Africa has relatively few registered choristers, we are arguably the greatest choral nation in the world. In African culture, most occasions are accompanied by four-part singing, and it is plausible to suggest that 40 million people or 90% of the population sing in a choir, be it formally or informally. HIV and AIDS has become an even bigger challenge, and it seems only natural that this scourge should also be fought through song and dance. By utilising a choir to spread HIV and AIDS awareness messages, we tap into one of Africa's greatest recourses and spread the awareness campaign to the audience in an enjoyable and understandable way.

According to the *SouthAfrica.Info*[4] website, sport is the national religion: "Transcending race, politics or language group, sport unites the country, and not just the male half of it. When a South African team wins, a cacophony of hooting, cheering, banging of dustbin lids, trumpeting on cow horns and fireworks reverberates across the largest cities. The national adrenaline goes into overdrive. Maybe even the Gross Domestic Product (GDP) goes up. Just don't look too cheerful on the Monday morning after a dismal sporting weekend! Sport, like no other South African institution, has shown it has the power to heal old wounds. When the Springboks won the Rugby World Cup on home turf in 1995, Nelson Mandela donned the No 6 shirt of the team's captain - François Pienaar, a white Afrikaner - and the two embraced in a spontaneous gesture of racial reconciliation which melted hearts around the country." Football – or soccer, as we call it – is the most widely played sport in South Africa, with its traditional support base in the black community. For many South Africans the country's proudest sporting moment came when it won the African Nations Cup on home turf in 1996 and got the right to bid for 2010 FIFA World Cup. Soccer is intensely followed, and the quality of the local game keeps improving, as demonstrated by the increasing number of South African players-in-exile among the glamorous European clubs. Local teams, organized in a national league plus a plethora of knock-out cups, are followed with passion by paint-daubed, costumed, whistling and cheering fans. The Vuvuzelas are part of South African soccer-loving culture. The nation-building power of sport, first through the rugby match between the Stormers and the Blue Bulls in the Orlando Stadium, and the powerful bonding of South Africans in supporting the Bafana Bafana team, as well as them demonstrating the pride in their country via mirror socks, flags on the cars, and flags on their homes and businesses, has been one of the most wonderful benefits of the World Cup, and is likely to last well beyond the end of the World Cup. The "gees" Ke Nako that was the theme of the World Cup grew throughout the World Cup into an unheard of spirit of national pride, surpassing that of the Rugby World Cup in 1995. Not only at a local level has the 2010 FIFA World Cup given South Africans an inside into each others' world. It has also shown to the world that through sports we can establish an environment of better understanding, better dialogue with less violence and less crime

The problem, however, is that there is hardly a national sports policy that capitalises on this potential. The national organizing committee of the 2010 World Cup was so heavily involved in arranging the event that they hardly spent time or energy on developing a local infrastructure for soccer with adequate training facilities, schooling of coaches and trainers, production of training manuals, etc. Anyway, soccer organizations of Western countries perceive it as their task to offer local sport clubs, local schools and NGOs their help in the development of training facilities, training methods, etc. They provide these local clubs with money for contracts for soccer players, trainers and organizers. It proved that the local sport authorities have difficulty handling this – relatively wealthy – situation. This Western support will probably only last during the period that the soccer world is caught up in the fever of the 2010 World Cup, but when this mood is gone, the sponsors withdraw, leaving behind a technically, mentally and financially underdeveloped soccer infrastructure (Milikowski & Hoekstra, 2009). This is a missed opportunity for the development of young talent in an underdeveloped environment. Nevertheless, the mental and organizational impetus caused by the 2010 World Cup in South Africa has to be used on a local level to develop a soccer infrastructure for youth.

In order to present an Asset-Based Community Development (ABCD) programme to a community that utilises Sports, Arts & Culture as a driver to investigate, assess and develop the potential present, requires infrastructure. The Ndlovu Care Group established a quality sports complex inside the township through donor funding, consisting of a 6x6 soccer field, tennis court, two volleyball fields, a basketball field, a netball field and a complete community indoor centre with a gymnasium and halls to accommodate the local boxing club, the aerobics classes, the ballroom dancers, etc.

For music, drama and other cultural events, Ndlovu Care Group erected 'The Miracle', a township amphitheatre with 1,000 seats, a proper stage with first-class equipment. It offers an open air cinema, indoor space for ballet and dance classes, rooms for music tutorials on individual instruments, etc.

A training centre to develop computer literacy amongst the employees of Ndlovu Care Group developed over time into a computer school with internet access for the community. This institute is now a sustainable business providing education for the community as a whole.

Statements like "Second best is good enough for Africa" should be treated with the disgust it deserves. It demands creative investment to develop structures like those described above, but if we calculate the return on the financial investment, then this is a sound investment in social capital. The benefit of this programme is that talent already present in the community gets the opportunity to develop in a professional manner, this creates opportunities people can benefit from to advance in life, a chance the system they were raised in forgot to offer them.

2. Target Groups

The target groups for the Sport, Art, Culture, and Life Skills (motivation) programmes are the inhabitants of the demarcated rural areas where the Rural Advancement Plan is implemented. The target groups are segmented according to demographics, psychographics, and sociographics and referred to specific development programmes, viz. sport, music, art, life skills, and academic programmes, depending on their needs, talents, and abilities. Specific target groups include: schools, those talented in sport and music (including persons with a disability), orphans and vulnerable children, individuals enrolled in lifelong and long-term treatment programmes (HIV & AIDS, TB, chronic diseases), the youth, school pupils who need academic support.

The overall objective of all the Rural Advancement Plan programmes is to contribute to the primary prevention of poverty and its by-products, and to retain the community within the programmes. This is achieved through educating children/ youth in and out of school on a variety of learning areas and life skills, to enrich their lives and to support them in becoming and staying empowered, healthy, and fulfilled.

The motivation programmes also promote the participation of the target groups in support groups where they learn and get more involved in activities that benefit themselves and their communities, and where they compete and gain exposure. The programmes provide developmentally appropriate opportunities for people to nurture skills and talents, practise these until they are learned, and be able to use them as necessary throughout a lifetime. Through the experiential learning process, youth internalize the knowledge and gain the ability to apply the skills appropriately. The youth clubs provide more opportunities for participation than traditional classroom learning. The clubs can be more fun for youth where, for example, they are involved in games, drama & dance, and sporting competitions on specific issues. Being in clubs helps youth develop leadership skills and assists them in determining their own priorities in life. Youth can be powerful advocates (ambassadors) for change among their peers, family members and the wider community. Belonging in the different groups also creates a sense of security, safety and control over one's life. Another major benefit is the development of group cohesiveness and consequent peer group support. The group is the primary learning and support vehicle for the participants. This ensures that when participants leave the programme, they have an ongoing and effective support network.

Once the youth complete their secondary schooling, school leavers need preparation for an employable future and economic success. The motivation programmes enhance employment and income-earning opportunities (small business development) of unemployed youth through training courses and internship placement opportunities facilitated by the CHAMP programme.

3. Aims

The Motivation programme aims to promote opportunities for people to develop their potential through sport, music, academics (support with their schoolwork), and a life skills programme with initiatives to:
– improve health;
– encourage social cohesion; and
– regenerate communities, reduce teenage pregnancies and HIV infections.

CHAMP interventions are not only about increasing the number of participants in the different activities; they are also about improving capacity:
- increasing confidence and belief in self and others;
- developing skills;
- providing equal opportunities; and
- contributing to the overall good of the community.

The Motivation programme wants to ensure that:
- there are opportunities for people to maximise their potential through sport, music and life skills;
- people in rural areas have the opportunity to lead a tolerable life while also improving their skills;
- young people are further enabled and not deprived of the opportunity inherent in their potential and capabilities to secure a future and to enjoy life;
- young people have a sense of belonging.

3.1. Sport Programme

The goals of this programme are to:
- empower the most disadvantaged persons with and without a disability in South Africa;
- improve the quality of their lives through education (sport) and participation;
- increase personal and social awareness with and for disabled people through sport and movement as instruments to develop self-esteem;
- identify, develop, and guide sporting talent to lead to employable careers;
- teach sporting rules, regulations, and train sporting coaches and referees.

3.2. Life Skills Programme

This programme attempts to:
- develop and promote a healthy self-concept and self-image of identified orphaned and vulnerable children, youth, and community members;
- improve coping skills, self-esteem, self-confidence, self-actualisation and mobilisation;
- promote sense of belonging, sense of security, social integration and emotional stability;
- unlock and develop existing potential and talents;
- improve their learning ability and academic achievement - graduate from school; and
- prevent school dropouts.

3.3. Ndlovu Music Academy (NMA)

The township amphitheatre houses the music programmes offered to the community:

- through music education; the Ndlovu Music Academy aims to identify, grade, develop, and nurture music skills within the local community, which will result in employment within the music industry, unearth and develop local traditional music, and promote the HIV and AIDS awareness programmes of the NCG;
- the NMA teaches music lessons on the piano and other instruments to expand the individuals' reference framework and enhances cultural development;
- regular performances expose the community to art & cultural performance and the choristers to the outside world: e.g. the Ndlovu Youth Choir, part of the NMA, has shared the stage with some of Tshwane's top choirs;
- All choristers are enrolled for music theory with the Royal school of music in London.

Future plans include:
- Quality individual music tuition that includes music theory. The programme will first look to offer employment to good qualified music teachers from the community. If we are unable to find suitable teachers, we will have to attract good teachers outside our community to give lessons. Lessons will initially only include theory, piano and voice. As the programme progresses, we aim to offer lessons in various instruments on request from the community. This would include jazz instruments as well as classical instruments. For older students lessons will be offered in a stimulating manner different to the traditional music education models. For example, a young child would learn simple folk tunes, and adults would be fast-tracked to jazz and popular music.
- Publish a book on traditional African folk tunes which will help make the lessons relevant, as well as promote traditional African music, which is fast losing ground to popular music such as hip-hop (Kwaito) and house music.
- Instrument lessons will be presented to children of five years and older, and progress will be regularly monitored through internal and external examinations as well as performances. The Instrument Tuition will be embedded in the NCG AIDS Awareness Programme, the NCG Child Care Programme and the Life Skills Training Programme, but it will also be open to members from the community.
- 'Umntwana Umculo' (Children's Music) will be a programme based on similar, successful, children's music education programmes. Like all other Ndlovu programmes, it will be presented with a strong African theme. It will be offered to children between six months and five years old. It will aim to nurture a child's cognitive, emotional, social, language, and early physical development through music. The programme will include extensive ensemble work that will develop the children's confidence with singing and speaking and will support scholastic achievement. This will encourage a child to discover an engaging musical world while building confidence, self-control, and communication skills. Listening and taking turns encourages blossoming social skills. 'Umntwana Umculo' will provide age-appropriate musical experiences that lead children towards an appreciation of the many colours, sounds and emotions that music evokes. It will create a learning environment that integrates music, expressive language, peer and parent interaction and play, whilst encouraging the building of characteristics related to successful learning in later school education; self-confidence, self-expression, social skills

and cooperation. This will be presented in conjunction with the Ndlovu Pre-Schools in Ntwane, Thabachabedu, Phooko and Marapong.

- The African drumming ensemble will be linked with traditional dancing classes. Performers will wear traditional costumes manufactured by the community and will be directed by one of the local residents. They will not only perform at the theatre but at various community functions, celebrations and HIV and AIDS awareness campaigns.

3.4. Cultural Activities

These activities aim at:
- promoting mass participation in arts and culture activities, cultural heritage and mainstreaming its role in socio-economic development;
- building the capacity in the target communities to develop employable skills and maximise talent.

The following disciplines are used:
- Craft: Making craft products and developing a craft outlet, e.g. ceramics, pottery, wood carving, embroidery, tapestry, bead-making, weaving and textile design, building on existing community skills.
- Dance and choreography: Various dance performances with a preference for local traditional dances.
- Literature: Story-telling, reading and poetry writing to capture folklore and myths for future generations, to be published in a book.
- Multi-discipline: Community arts and cultural events and community arts festivals.
- Theatre and musical theatre: Script writing, performances, story-telling, puppetry and musical theatre.
- Visual arts: Drawing and painting.

4. Assessment of the Starting Position of the Target Groups

The Asset-Based Community Development (ABCD) approach views communities as entities with existing functional systems that are arranged to the benefit of the communities. Communities have strong networks that already exist but might not be visible to an outsider. The ABCD approach embraces the political, civil society, faith-based, and cultural networks already in the community to launch development initiatives from.

At the individual level, the ABCD approach views people as positive actors in their lives and communities. It sees investing in talented people as a significant opportunity to harness their potential to improve individual achievement, which contributes to the wealth of the community. ABCD focuses on the positive contributions people can make with the assets that they already possess rather than the ones they are lacking. Within this context, people with potential need to be supported to engage positively and effectively in their community's development through target-friendly education emphasizing the importance of participation, life skills and livelihood development, and access to a variety of structured opportunities for civic engagement appropriate for these people's individual interests, goals, and skill sets.

Segmentation of the community into targets that fit into specific motivation programmes forms the basis of the success of the approach as the incumbents are talented, and achievement comes naturally.

4.1. Sport Programme

The sport grounds include a soccer field, tennis courts, netball, basketball, and volleyball courts, and a fully equipped gymnasium. The programme identifies and nurtures sporting talent and develops the talent at individual or team levels:
- qualified fitness instructors design personal training programmes for individuals attending the gymnasium;
- qualified coaches offer sport coaching weekly in tennis, soccer, and netball;
- running club trains long-distance runners.
- qualified fitness instructors offer personal training in the gymnasium as a rehabilitation centre for disabled people or recovering AIDS patients who are in need of physical stimulation and exercise.

4.2. Life Skills Programme

The life skills programme arranges after school activities and assistance with homework for school-going children in the area at the sports grounds. The programme provides the children with entertainment, social integration and academic stimulation:
- orphans and vulnerable children attend life skills training workshops daily after school at the sport grounds under supervision of Life Skills trainers;
- through cooperation with local schools, children's academic progress and achievement are monitored and supported when needed;
- CHAMP is starting a Saturday Academy to support children from child-headed households with academic progress;
- Life Skills trainers utilise Life Skills Orientation periods in local schools to create awareness, destigmatise, and mobilise the school-going youth.

4.3. Ndlovu Music Academy

Through music education the Ndlovu Music Academy (NMA) identifies, grades, develops, and nurtures skills within the local community, which results in improved individual and group self-esteem, and hopefully employment within the music industry. The NMA unearths and develops local traditional music and promotes the HIV and AIDS awareness messages of the Rural Advancement Plan. The NMA is located at The Miracle theater, which was made possible by donations from sponsors in the Netherlands who recognised the importance of the arts, and the role the arts and specifically music plays in the prevention of disease, alleviation of poverty, sustainable social transformation, and the uplifting of individuals through talent identification and nurturing. All music programmes aim to develop community-based musical skills whilst providing an underprivileged community with excellent entertainment and a form of escapism from the social ills of an impoverished society. Music lessons incorporate traditional music with Western teaching methodology in order to be relevant as well as preserving the cultural identity of the community.

The NMA established a youth choir (age 13-24) as this is the most effective way of introducing the NMA to the community. NMA also started a conductor-training programme, which includes the Associated Board of the Royal School of Music (UK) music theory examinations. The NMA offers quality individual music tuition to a community that has seldom been exposed to development through education in art and cultural programmes due to its isolated geographical location. Lessons will initially only include music theory, piano and voice. As the programme progresses and partnerships with donors are established, NMA will expand with lessons in various instruments on request from the community. This would include jazz instruments as well as classical instruments and a brass band.

Future plans include a brass band, jazz programmes, a book on traditional songs and stories, drama, and dance lessons.

5. Working Methods

The future of rural communities depends upon productive, positive, and prepared youth. Preparing today's youth to be healthy, well-educated, involved, and capable of leadership signifies a strong and secure future. Also, by addressing the root issues of the HIV and AIDS pandemic amongst youth, the programme achieves specific developmental outcomes through ABCD. Thus, the CHAMP motivation programme assists by creating a positive and enabling platform, focusing on the following:
- promoting and developing skills and abilities to support recreation, leisure, and physical well-being;
- preparing youth for an employable future and economic success;
- developing personal competency skills: self-confidence and self-awareness, decision-making, personal responsibility, personal accountability for actions, selecting positive peers, and avoiding risky behaviours;
- developing interpersonal skills: teamwork, leading and serving others (community service and leadership skills), relationship and communication (communication skills, conflict management skills);
- developing marketable skills: career choices, planning and computer literacy; and
- retaining individuals in developmental programmes for as long as the need arises and the person is prepared for a normalised life with job perspective and self-care.

Ndlovu Care Group identified talent and skills development as an essential part of rural advancement in the CHAMP programme. The objective of CHAMP is to find and build on local talent, skills, and abilities, and develop these to create champions from the community. These champions will embody a future orientation for the individuals and the community, and the individuals will be much better equipped to exploit job opportunities in their areas of ability. The CHAMP Sport, Art and Culture programmes follow a similar approach to assist with the development of sport and academic ability. Not only do the participants of the programme benefit, but the entire community of Elandsdoorn will benefit from the music produced at the NMA through performances in the theatre and interactive HIV and AIDS awareness programmes and poverty alleviation programmes. Skills are developed and appreciated, and this increases the social capital of all the participants and their families, which in turn creates jobs and an influx of money into the community. This eventually uplifts the entire community through breaking the vicious cycle of poverty and the associated lack of opportunity in rural communities, and contributes towards community cohesion.

The CHAMP Motivation programme equips individuals with skills and attitudes supportive of developing positive futures and lifelong learning. As a departure point, these individuals require an understanding of self as the basis for healthy interactions with others, for career development, and for lifelong learning. They also require a safe and caring school and community environment in which to explore ideas and issues surrounding personal choice, to seek accurate information, and to practise healthy behaviour. Developing their life skills involves teaching them about the habits, behaviours, interactions and decisions related to healthy daily living and planning for the future. It is personal in nature and involves developing abilities based on a body of knowledge and practice that builds on personal values and beliefs within the context of family, school and community.

The programme identifies talents and skills to motivate children and youth towards developing skills and abilities. All NCG programmes create awareness, and refer talented individuals to appropriate programmes. The objective is to develop each individual kid according to his own potential to achieve self-actualisation and hopefully employment or further study in that field.

5.1. Sport Programme

James Humphrey[5] (2003; p. 4) states in his book *Child Development through Sports* that experimental evidence has shown that a human being must be considered as a whole and not a collection of parts. This means that a child is a unified individual, or what is more commonly known as the *whole* child. The Ndlovu sports programme applies this comprehensive approach in its sport programme too, according to the RAP continuum of care for prevention and motivation; the children's needs are addressed to prevent disability and developmental problems, and then they are motivated to build on their strengths to achieve whole-child well-being.

Humphrey states further that total development encompasses the various major forms of development. All of these components – physical, social, emotional, and intellectual – are highly interrelated and interdependent. All are of importance to well-being. Humphrey continues: 'The condition of any one of these forms of development affects all other forms to a degree and, thus, development as a whole. When a nervous child stutters or becomes nauseated, a mental state is not necessarily causing a physical symptom. On the contrary, a pressure imposed upon the child causes a series of reactions, which includes thought, verbalization, digestive processes, and muscular function. It is not always true that the mind causes the body to become upset by a particular situation and reflects its upset in several ways, including disturbances in thought, feeling, and bodily processes. The whole child responds to the social and physical environment, and as he or she is affected by the environment, the child in turn has an effect upon it. However, since physical *or* intellectual development, rather than physical *and* intellectual development, has been glorified, we divide the two in our minds' (Humphrey, 2003; p. 4).

The same source states: 'Health is now being considered more and more in terms of *well-being*, which is perhaps our most important human value. Considering health in terms of absence of disease places it in a negative sense. The well-being concept places positive emphasis on the term. It seems logical to assume that modern society's goal should be directed towards achieving the highest level of well-being for all of its citizens' (p. 15). Humphrey describes health as a triangle of: (1) nutrition and diet, (2) rest and sleep, and (3) physical activity and exercise.

Through normalisation of the development and disabilities that exist in the children and visitors to the sport grounds, the programme builds strong and balanced individuals, through motivation, who are ready to utilise their potential.

5.2. The Life Skills Programme

In his book *Man's search for meaning*, Viktor Frankl (1962) shares his philosophy on life. He called this philosophy 'logotherapy', and it is based on a spiritual survival mechanism he developed in World War II while interred in a concentration camp. He believes that his spiritual survival led to his physical survival, and this allowed him to survive the war. Frankl believes that you cannot avoid suffering or challenges in life; it is what you choose to make of them that is important. Frankl states that to find meaning in adversity and to move forward with a new purpose in life, you need a 'big enough WHY, then you could do any HOW'. The existential aspect of Frankl's psychotherapy maintains man always has the ability to choose; no matter the biological, or environmental forces. An important aspect of this therapy is known as the "tragic triad": pain, guilt, and death. Frankl's "Case for a Tragic Optimism" uses this philosophy to demonstrate... "optimism in the face of tragedy and in view of the human potential, which at its best always allows for". The Life Skills programme motivates children to make the best of their environment and abilities, and exposes them to alternatives that might be available for them to lead a responsible and productive life. The programme debriefs children and provides them with tools and development programmes to rise above the negative aspects of their environment and then to build on their strengths to compete for opportunities.

"Freedom is not the last word; freedom is only part of the story and half of the truth. The positive aspect of freedom is responsibleness... That is why I recommend that the Statue of Liberty on the East Coast be supplemented by a Statue of Responsibility on the West Coast" (Warnock, 2005).

5.3. The Music Academy

A Music Director oversees the NMA, whose responsibilities include project development, performances, community consultations, teacher recruiting, standard evaluation, local and international liaison, group directing and skills development. A Logistics Manager from the community assists the director, arranging rehearsal and lesson schedules, transport, clothing, logistics and other necessities. S/he reports matters regarding the programme to the director on a daily basis. S/he is an internal appointment from the CHAMP Prevention programme and receives training in theatre management through a bursary at a theatre in Berlin.

The Choral Programme is embedded in the CHAMP Prevention, the Children's, and the Life Skills Training programmes. The choir's repertoire not only consists of HIV and AIDS awareness messages but incorporates many of South Africa's various musical genres. A strong emphasis is placed on preserving traditional music and ensuring its longevity.

The choir performs acapella music as well as songs accompanied by a band. As the programme progresses, the professional musicians brought in to accompany the choir at important events will be replaced by local musicians who will have hopefully acquired their skills from the Ndlovu Music Programme. The aim is eventually to establish children's choirs (2-5 years old) and (6-13 years old), an adult choir and a staff choir, in addition to the youth choir (13-24 years old). The NMA choral programme also includes conductor training and formal music theory training.

The advantages of music and music education are undeniable. The Children's Music Workshop[6] website identifies the following twelve benefits:

1. Early musical training helps develop brain areas involved in language and reasoning. Recent studies have clearly indicated that musical training physically develops the part of the left side of the brain known to be involved with processing language, and can actually wire the brain's circuits in specific ways. Linking familiar songs to new information can also help imprint information on young minds.

2. There is also a causal link between music and spatial intelligence (the ability to perceive the world accurately and to form mental pictures of things). This kind of intelligence, by which one can visualize various elements that should go together, is critical to the sort of thinking necessary for everything from solving advanced mathematics problems to being able to pack a book-bag with everything that will be needed for the day.

3. Students of the arts learn to think creatively and to solve problems by imagining various solutions, rejecting outdated rules and assumptions. Questions about the arts do not have only one right answer.

4. Recent studies show that students who study the arts are more successful on standardized tests such as the Scholastic Assessment Test (SAT).[7] They also achieve higher grades in high school.

5. A study of the arts provides children with an internal glimpse of other cultures and teaches them to be empathetic towards the people of these cultures. This development of compassion and empathy, as opposed to the development of greed and a 'me first' attitude, provides a bridge across cultural chasms that leads to respect for other races at an early age.

6. Students of music learn craftsmanship as they study how details are painstakingly put together and what constitutes good, as opposed to mediocre, work. These standards, when applied to a student's own work, demand a new level of excellence and require students to tap their inner resources.

7. In music, a mistake is a mistake; the instrument is in tune or not, the notes are well played or not, the entrance is made or not. It is only by much hard work that

a successful performance is possible. Through music study, students learn the value of sustained effort to achieve excellence and the concrete rewards of hard work.

8. Music study enhances teamwork skills and discipline. In order for an orchestra to sound good, all players must work together harmoniously towards a single goal, the performance, and must commit to learning music, attending rehearsals, and practising.

9. Music provides children with a means of self-expression. Now that there is relative security in the basics of existence, the challenge is to make life meaningful and to reach for a higher stage of development. Everyone needs to be in touch at some point in life with their core, with what they are and what they feel. Self-esteem is a by-product of this self-expression.

10. Music study develops skills that are necessary in the workplace. It focuses on "doing" as opposed to observing, and teaches students how to perform, literally, anywhere in the world.

11. Employers are looking for multi-dimensional workers with the sort of flexible and supple intellects that music education helps to create as described above. In the music classroom, students can also learn to communicate better and cooperate with one another.

12. Music performance teaches young people to conquer fear and to take risks. A little anxiety is a good thing, and something that will occur often in life. Dealing with it early often makes it less of a problem later. Risk-taking is essential if a child is to fully develop his or her potential.

An arts education exposes children to the incomparable. Exposing children to a comprehensive music and art education opens up a world to them that is not available in mainstream syllabi. Children need deliberate training in art, music, and culture to develop holistically.

5.4. The Relationship Between Aims and Working Methods

In the programme evaluation we discern between specific effects or outcomes and non-specific effects of an intervention. Specific effects are the intended outcomes, non-specific effects are the unintended, or additional, or incidental outcomes. For example, the specific effect of learning to play the piano is the technical and musical improvement of piano playing. A non-specific effect could be that the progress in piano playing contributes to the enhancement of self-esteem and the general feeling of competency of the child who is learning to play.

If a programme has to fulfil several different aims, in other words has several intended goals, these goals only could be attained by means of activities specifically designed to achieve specific goals, For example, sport could contribute to physical well-being, self-confidence, social awareness, etc. A specific goal of a sport activity can only be reached when the sport activities to be carried out are carefully designed for that specific aim. In other words: having a NCG sport programme does not mean that all the intended goals will be realised. From a scientific point of view, we could say that the internal validity of a programme is high when there is proven evidence that the working methods of a specific programme are directly related to a specific aim of the programme (Cohen, Manion & Morrison, 2000). It's the task of an NGO like NCG to develop manuals for each CHAMP programme, in which the planned and proven relationship between the different aspects of that programme are described.

6. Evaluation

NCC has a comprehensive monitoring and evaluation (M&E) action plan. The plan is meant to ensure that NCG programmes under the RAP:
1. are doing the right things in the right way and that their activities are achieving real benefits for the individual and the community;
2. gather high-quality data that can be used for strategic decision-making and programme improvement; and
3. are making the most efficient use of resources, and that its programmes are relevant to the needs of the communities.

Process indicators are continually reviewed, and the staff measure targets they set for themselves and agree with programme management. The staff also monitors the implementation of the activities. Monitoring is an essential activity because it helps identify gaps, challenges, and target group requirements, as well as assuring that these needs are being met by the implementing partners. NCG, through the M&E unit, provides M&E training to community partners and organisations to ensure that community structures are aligned with CHAMP objectives. By providing its partners with comprehensive M&E training, easy-to-use and up-to-date tools, NCG is providing organisations at a grassroots level with important skills to make a positive impact on the lives of rural inhabitants.

The M&E and Research Department regularly assist, consult and advise the Programme Management Team on M&E-related matters. The M&E follows the logical framework approach, which outlines objectives, indicators for measuring success, and a comprehensive monitoring and evaluation plan. Indicators of achievement for outputs, outcomes and goals, and a plan for M&E using those indicators, are outlined in the M&E plan for the Sport, Art and Culture Programme to depict the extent to which programme results are being or have been achieved (see also Chapter 4).

Attention is paid to both formative (process) monitoring and summative (product) evaluation. Both the efficiency of a process and the success of the outcomes are crucial in assessing the success of an intervention. Establishing whether we have met our stated outcomes will inform the formative/process evaluations for the programme. Summative/product success will be evaluated by reflecting upon the stated objectives of the programme and whether they have been met through the activities. Deriving from the M&E processes and their evaluation, improvements to the project will be suggested and research protocols formulated. Research will be conducted on an ongoing basis in cooperation with various institutions.

The M&E plan covers the following aspects:
- defining indicators, data sources, data collection methodologies, frequency of data collection, and who is responsible;
- establishing a baseline for the indicators.

The role of M&E would be to assist with:
- preparing monitoring forms;
- scheduling data collection and reporting;
- training staff and partner community organisations in monitoring;
- organising the information infrastructure (such as a paper filing system or computer database) and procedures for storing and reporting information;
- planning the flow of information to major partners;
- planning appropriate management action if performance targets are not met;
- planning for periodic checks on the accuracy of the information collected;
- performing quality assurance on an ongoing basis;
- evaluating planning, progress and results against the set objectives, standards and indicators, and reporting these accordingly every month;
- organising regular meetings with the programme team and providing feedback on progress to the stakeholders to enhance the quality of the programme;
- incorporating staff capacity development in the planning to strengthen the programme.

The following factors ensure the sustainability of the programme:
- developing a model that works closely with the government that the government can adopt after a specific time-frame;
- strengthening the system to increase and maintain the number of people participating in arts and culture activities;
- diversifying funding sources.

Notes

1. Benjamin Disraeli (21 December 1804 – 19 April 1881), British prime minister, parliamentarian, Conservative statesman and literary figure. Available from: http://www.quotationspage.com/quotes/Benjamin_Disraeli
2. http://www.answers.com/topic/awareness-interest-desire-action-aida
3. http://www.edpsycinteractive.org/topics/regsys/maslow.html
4. http://www.southafrica.info/about/sport/sportsa.htm
5. James H. Humphrey, EdD, Professor Emeritus, Department of Kinesiology, University of Maryland
6. http://www.childrenmusicworkshop.com
7. The SAT test is the benchmark test that potential American college students take every year. The SAT test is administered by the College Board, which claims that it is the best method to judge if a student has the right aptitude to enter college. Available from: http://sattestinfo.net/

References

Centre for Higher Education and Transformation (CHET) and the Further Education and Training Institute (FETI) (2009). *Responding to the educational needs of post-school youth – determining the scope of the problem and developing a capacity-building model. First Draft Synthesis Report June 2009.* Wynberg: CHET.

Cohen, L., Manion, L. & Morrison, K. (2000). *Research Methods in Education.* New York/London: RoutledgeFalmer.

Frankl, V. (1962). *Man's search for meaning: An introduction to logotherapy.* Boston: Beacon Press.

Herzberg, F., Mausner, B. & Snyderman, B.(1959). *The motivation to work.* New York: Wiley.

Humphrey, J.H. (2003). *Child Development through Sports.* New York: The Haworth Press, Inc.

Kotler, P. & Lee N. (2009). *Up and Out of Poverty: The Social Marketing Solution.* Upper Saddle River, New Jersey: Wharton School Publishing-Pearson.

Milikowski, F. & Hoekstra, E. (2009). *De droom van Zuid-Afrika. Achter de schermen bij het WK 2010.* Amsterdam: Uitgeverij Carrera.

Prahalad, C.K. (2005). *The Fortune at the Bottom of the Pyramid: Eradicating Poverty through Profits.* Upper Saddle River, NJ: Wharton School Publishing-Pearson.

Rothman A. (2000). Toward a theory based analysis of behavioural maintenance. *Health Psychology, 9*, 64–9.

Seligman, M. (2003). *Authentic Happiness: Using the New Positive Psychology to Realise Your Potential for Lasting Fulfilment.* London/Boston: Nicholas Brealy publishing.

Shisana, O., Rehle, T., Simbayi, L., Zuma, K., Jooste, S., Pillay-van-Wyk, V., Mbelle, N., Van Zyl, J., Parker, W., Zungu, N., Pezi, S. & the SABSSM III Implementation Team (2008). *South African National HIV Prevalence, Incidence, Behaviour and Communication Survey, 2008. A Turning Tide Among Teenagers?* HSRC Press: Public Health.

Smith, S. C. (2005). *Ending Global Poverty: A guide to what works.* New York: Palgrave-MacMillan.

United Nations (2006). *The Millennium Development Goals Report.* New York: UNO.

Warnock, C. (2005). *If freedom is to endure, liberty must be joined with responsibility. "Statue of Responsibility".* Utah: Daily Herald.

Weiser, S., Wolfe, W., Kebaabetswe, P., Makhema, J., Dickenson, D., Mompati, K., Sherif, M., Tlou, S., Moffat, H., Onen, C., Hensle, K., Thior, I. & Marlink, R. (2002). Determinants of antiretroviral treatment adherence among patients with HIV and AIDS in Botswana. International Conference on AIDS. *Int Conf AIDS, 7-12,* 14: abstract no. WePeB5851.

Epilogue

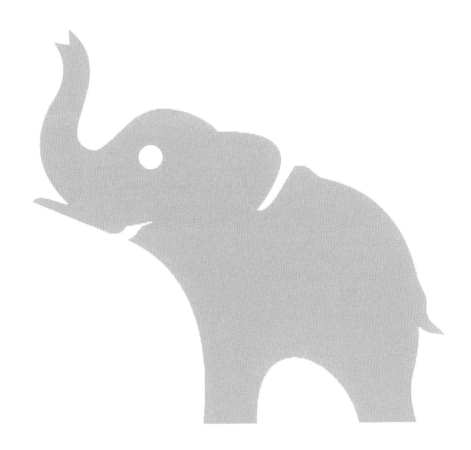

AIDS Prevention Programmes in Southern Africa: Applying Western Knowledge and Technology in Local Cultures[1]

Frank Miedema[a]

The great news at the AIDS Conference in Vancouver in 1996 was that an effective anti-HIV treatment had finally been found. For the first time, AIDS and HIV could be halted by medication, and HIV had become a normal, treatable, infectious disease. For many years, people had been waiting for a real breakthrough in the fight against AIDS as the epidemic was spreading like wildfire throughout Africa, and it was expected that the virus would take the same course in the densely populated areas of Thailand, Indonesia, India, Brazil and China. It was already recognized that HIV was spreading in a completely different way in Africa than it was in the USA and Europe. There were numerous signs that heterosexuals were rapidly becoming infected in Africa, whereas the infection was still restricted to the classic high-risk groups in Europe and the USA, i.e. homosexual males and drug users. No-one could really understand why HIV was spreading indiscriminately through all the various population groups in developing countries. The high percentage of rural women who were infected with HIV despite seeming to have a single regular partner was particularly strange. The American sociologist, Martina Morris, collaborated with Mirjam Kretzschmar, a German epidemiologist working in the Netherlands, on an epidemiological-mathematical model that could explain the rapid spread of the HIV epidemic in Africa (Morris & Kretzschmar, 1997). As so often happens in science, the idea went unnoticed for some time, but it is now increasingly being seen as a very important contribution towards our understanding of the HIV epidemic. In 2004, in the medical journal *The Lancet* and in the *New York Times*, two American researchers – Halperin and Epstein – put Morris and Kretzschmar's '*concurrent partnership*' hypothesis forward as the only plausible explanation for the high-speed spread of HIV and AIDS in southern Africa. They called for the use of this hypothesis as a basis for the development of prevention campaigns that could be effective in countries such as Botswana and South Africa. One of the authors of the article in *The Lancet* was Helen Epstein, who in 2007 wrote a compelling book entitled cryptically, '*The invisible cure: Africa, the West and the fight against AIDS*' (Epstein, 2007). That book tells the story of the AIDS epidemic in various countries in southeast Africa, with particular emphasis on South Africa, Botswana, Mozambique and Uganda, and follows up on the Western world's reaction and its AIDS prevention programmes; it comes to

a. Professor of Immunology and Dean, University Medical Centre Utrecht, the Netherlands

the shocking conclusion that those programmes, which cost many billions of dollars, are often ineffective because they are conceived against the background of Western knowledge and culture and have too little affinity with the local cultural situation.

The AIDS prevention programmes were aimed at the use of condoms and combatting STDs. Preaching monogamy and abstinence to groups such as prostitutes, who display high-risk behaviour, while trying to involve the entire population in the programmes proved to be pointless. Despite the increasing use of condoms and the inordinately costly campaigns, vast numbers of ordinary men and women, from rich to poor, high class to low class, were still succumbing to AIDS. Usable research data were lacking, but speculation was rife: the situation was thought to be the result of widespread promiscuity, poverty, poor hygiene, the effect of STDs and even the different forms of exotic blood rituals practised in Africa. Seen in retrospect, our ideas about the rapid spread of HIV in southern Africa took shape only slowly. We were apparently missing some essential piece of knowledge about the sexual customs in southern Africa. Martina Morris was carrying out sociological research in Uganda, and during a visit to Kampala in 1993 she was put on the trail of this missing link. Like so many people since, Morris was able to establish that, on average, Africans have just as many sexual partners during their lifetimes as heterosexual men and women in Europe do. Surprisingly, though, she found that quite a large proportion of the men – and women, too – maintained simultaneous, stable and long-term sexual relations with two or even three different but regular partners. This was something that was traditionally considered to be perfectly normal in southern Africa. The 'concurrent partnership' hypothesis immediately illuminates how quickly HIV can spread in a population that includes a high level of such partnerships involving both men and women. Everyone is literally connected to everyone else, and if the virus is introduced into the network by an incautious person, it can rapidly infect everyone, even those who are themselves monogamous. The brief but acute infection period following HIV transmission provides the virus with the opportunity to spread like wildfire through a network, as for that brief period, there is a cascade of highly infectious persons within the network. In a population in which people are primarily serially monogamous, as in most Western and Asian countries, the virus becomes 'entombed' in those monogamous partnerships.

Given that insight, the failure of the prevention campaigns in southeast Africa is understandable. They were aimed at risk groups as defined by Western standards and overlooked the conventions of sexual relationships in countries such as Botswana and South Africa. As Epstein wrote, AIDS prevention workers in those countries eventually came to the conclusion that they had been wrongly informed, with all the collateral consequences. There was an increase of condom use in the case of incidental or commercial sex, but the regular partners within a network knew each other and therefore did not use condoms. Southeast Africa is the only region where HIV has been able to spread so widely in the population, but it is also the only part of the world with a tradition of concurrent, long-term sexual relationships. The women in Islamic countries have far less social freedom and do not have the opportunity to participate in multiple sexual relationships. It has been suggested that circumcision plays a more important role, but since circumcision is relatively rare in the USA, Europe and Brazil, it cannot explain the limited spread of HIV in those regions. The hypothesis not only explains why HIV has spread differently in Africa than it has in the USA and Europe, it also explains why there have not been unmanageable epidemics in countries such as China, Indonesia, Brazil, Thailand and India.

In the meantime, researchers had been wondering why the prevalence of HIV in Uganda was steadily decreasing, in sharp contrast to surrounding countries. Studies into sexual behaviour had been carried out in Uganda in 1989 and in 1995, and they provided an ideal and unique opportunity to ascertain what principal changes in sexual behaviour had coincided with the decline of the spread of HIV. On the basis of these two studies, UNAIDS workers published an article in the *AIDS* journal in 1997 in which they concluded that while condom use had increased significantly, there had been no reduction in the number of concurrent sexual relationships. This was important epidemiological confirmation and therefore good news for the methods of the WHO and UNAIDS that had been tested in the Western world (Asiimwe-Okor, Opio, Musinguzi, et al., 1997). Epstein and others came across the report containing the raw data from the field studies in the WHO Global Programme on AIDS. Re-analysis produced a totally different conclusion than the one set out in the article in *AIDS*, namely that there had been a strong abrupt reduction in the number of concurrent partners but no increase in condom use (Stoneburner & Low-Beer, 2004; Green, Halperin, Nantulya, & Hogle, 2006). That behavioural change was largely due to the impact of the attitude and approach of the Ugandan government, which proved to be quite different from those prevalent in neighbouring countries. Since the mid-1980s, AIDS and HIV had been spoken of openly, and even at the personal level; this was possible since people in Uganda are not reticent about speaking of sexual matters. The subject was broached in daily radio campaigns, and it was explained to people attending community health centres that it could affect anyone, not only prostitutes or people with many different sexual contacts. The campaign was entitled 'Zero Grazing', and its motto was: 'keep to a single, regular partner'. It seems that UNAIDS simply overlooked the effect of the reduction in partner numbers. Research data are often interpreted from a predefined hypothesis, and researchers can on occasion be blind for quite some time to an unexpected effect or phenomenon that does not fit into the original template. Since 2004, Epstein writes, UNAIDS and other major programmes in southern Africa have finally been putting more emphasis on partner reduction.

Epstein takes a politically correct stance on the subject of the application of antiviral therapies in Africa. She maintains that it is more effective to prevent HIV infection passing from mother to child, for example, than to treat infected children, however distressing it may be to deny AIDS patients a therapy that might prolong their life by around three years. It is enough of a challenge to get relatively simple and cheap health care such as vaccinations for measles – a disease which kills half a million children every year – or antimalaria bed nets to patients. There are few areas, if any, in developing countries where there is an infrastructure suitable for the provision of what even in the Western world is seen as complex health care, such as the combination therapies needed to treat HIV. Without proper medical supervision, there are enormous and already demonstrable risks that strains of HIV will develop that are unresponsive to therapy; the effectiveness of the therapy itself will be reduced, while high-risk behaviour will persist as a result of the reduced sensitivity to risk. In addition, it has been acknowledged that these multi-million dollar programmes are severely disrupting an already fragile health care system in Africa, a system that is crucial to the fight against untold other diseases, many of them also highly infectious. The lack of an adequate medical infrastructure and the way the few well-trained medical personnel are being enticed away to better-paid positions elsewhere are further factors of the same problem.

In this respect, Epstein espouses William Easterly's recent disquieting analysis of the failure, particularly the damaging effects of foreign aid in general (Easterly, 2006). But their opinions are at odds with the ideas expressed by the economist Jeffrey Sachs in his 'The end of poverty', in which he says that it is up to our generation to resolve the problems of sickness and poverty, and to do it quickly (Sachs, 2005). According to Sachs, it is only a question of goodwill and money, for the technology is available. Other experts are frustrated that Sachs –convinced as ever that he is right – is thwarting years of work on established aid programmes set up carefully with the aid of the local population. Ensuring a structural and sustainable supply of antiviral HIV therapy and antimalaria bed nets, for an extended period, to those parts of Africa where the need is greatest is not just a matter of money.

The question of how aid should be managed in the public health sector is a topical issue for us, given the health care and community development projects carried out by NCG in Elandsdoorn in South Africa and the associated Ndlovu Research Consortium set up by Hugo Tempelman in collaboration with the Universities of Utrecht and Pretoria. In the context of the NCG projects, which have been successfully managed for more than fifteen years, modern medical practices have been implemented and scientific research carried out in a local, non-Western environment and based on the customs and needs of the local population. NCG's integrated approach and the associated scientific analyses (e.g. Barth, van der Meer, Hoepelman, et al., 2008; Vermeer & Tempelman, 2008; Tempelman & Vermeer, 2009) have attracted a lot of attention, and these data in fact formed the basis for a new model design (see this book). The holistic approach reflected in the Ndlovu Care Group Model has led to the development of similar projects, also operating under NCG management, in the form of a 'community franchise model'. When setting up a new project, a local needs assessment is carried out within the local community. This takes the form of baseline studies which are then extrapolated with the assistance of enthusiastic community members and donors. The project is then implemented under the management of NCG and in collaboration with the local provincial and national authorities.

Ndlovu Care Group in Elandsdoorn has established its model for integrated health, child and community care also in other sites of South Africa. This implies that the developed model could contribute to the advancement of similar resource-poor communities across the country. This book presents a model that can be shared with those working in the same fields and for the same causes in order to contribute towards closing the poverty and treatment gaps in South Africa.

Note

1. An earlier version of this contribution, entitled 'Abstinence, Be faithful, use a Condom', was published in *De Academische Boekengids, 2008, 67,* 19- 24.

References

Asiimwe-Okor, G., Opio, A.A., Musinguzi, J., Madraa, E., Tembo, G., & Carael, M. (1997). Change in sexual behaviour and decline in HIV infection among young pregnant women in urban Uganda. *AIDS, 11,* 1175.

Barth, R.E., van der Meer, J.T., Hoepelman, I.M., Schrooders, P.A., van de Vijver, D.A., Geelen, S.P., & Tempelman, H.A. (2008). Effectiveness of highly active antiretroviral therapy administered by general practitioners in rural South Africa. *European Journal of Clinical Microbiology & Infectious Diseases, 27*(10), 977-984.

Easterly, W. (2006). *The white man's burden. Why the West's efforts to aid the rest have done so much ill and so little good.* New York: The Penguin Press.

Epstein, H. (2007). *The invisible cure: Africa, the West, and the fight against AIDS.* Farrar, New York: Straus and Giroux.

Halperin, D.T., & Epstein, H. (2004). Concurrent sexual partnerships help to explain Africa's high HIV prevalence: implications for prevention. *The Lancet, 364,* 69.

Green, E.C., Halperin, D.T., Nantulya, V. & Hogle, J.A. (2006). Uganda's HIV prevention success: the role of sexual behavior change and the national response. *AIDS and Behavior 10,* 335.

Morris, M., & Kretzschmar, M. (1997). Concurrent partnerships and the spread of HIV. *AIDS, 11,* 641.

Sachs, J.D. (2005). *The end of poverty.* New York: Penguin books.

Stoneburner, R.L., & Low-Beer, D. (2004). Population-level HIV declines and behavioural risk avoidance in Uganda. *Science, 304,* 714.

Tempelman, H.A., & Vermeer, A. (2009). An AIDS awareness programme in a rural area of South Africa to promote participation in Voluntary Counselling and Testing. In: Lagerwerf, L., Boer, H., & Wasserman, H. (eds.) (2009). *Health Communication in Southern Africa: Engaging with Social and Cultural Diversity (pp. 241-260).* SAVUSA series. Amsterdam: Rozenberg Publishers/Unisa Press.

Vermeer, A., & Tempelman, H. (eds.) (2008). *Health Care in rural South Africa: An Innovative Approach.* Amsterdam: VU University Press.

Donors of Ndlovu Care Group

Anglo Coal	South Africa
Biblionef	Netherlands
Department of Health & Social Development	South Africa
Diep in die Berg	South Africa
Ekasi TV	South Africa
Eltingh & Haarhuis Tennis and Events	Netherlands
Energetix	Germany
Gebroeders Bosch Stichting	Netherlands
German Embassy	Germany
Impumeleo Award Trust	South Africa
Johan Cruyff Foundation	Netherlands
Johanna den Donck-Grote Stichting	Netherlands
Nelson Mandela Children's Fund	South Africa
Nelson Mandela Kinder Fonds-NL	Netherlands
MTN	South Africa
NCDO	Netherlands
Oranje Groene Kruis	Netherlands
Rens Joosen Foundation	Netherlands
Respo International	Netherlands
Right to Care (USAID/PEPFAR)	USA
Rotary International	South Africa
Royal Netherlands Embassy	Netherlands
Stichting Liberty	Netherlands
Stichting Ngwenya	Netherlands
Stichting Sonnevanck	Netherlands
Tempelman Stiftung	Germany
Tjommie Foundation	Netherlands
Virgin Unite	UK
Vodacom Foundation	South Africa
VSO	UK
Wilde Ganzen	Netherlands
WOS Teteringen	Netherlands
Zorg voor Elandsdoorn	Netherlands

And all other donors who are involved in the Ndlovu Care Projects